# Effect Of Add On Yoga Therapy On Social Cognition In Schizophrenia

By:

**Dr. G Ramajayam**

**LIST OF ABBREVIATIONS USED**
(In alphabetical Order)

1. AS - Attributional styles
2. CPZ – Chlorpromazine
3. EEG – Electro-Encephalogram
4. ER - Emotion recognition
5. ER Index - Emotion Recognition Index
6. FOT Index - First Order Theory Of Mind Index
7. FPCI - Faux Pas Composite Index
8. fNIRS – functional Near Infrared Spectroscopy
9. MINI – Mini International Neuropsychiatric Interview
10. MNA - Mirror neuron activity
11. NC – Neuro-Cognition
12. RCT – Randomized Controlled Trial
13. RMANOVA – Repeated Measures Analysis of Variance
14. SANS - Scale for the Assessment of Negative Symptoms
15. SAPS- Scale for the Assessment of Positive Symptoms
16. SC - Social cognition
17. SCCS - Social Cognition Composite Score
18. SCRT - Social Cue Recognition Test
19. SCZ – Schizophrenia
20. SD – Standard Deviation
21. SOCRATIS - Social Cognition Rating Tool in Indian Setting
22. SoCueReTI - Social Cue Recognition Test in Indian Setting
23. SOT Index - Second Order Theory Of Mind Index

24. SP - Social perception
25. TMS - Transcranial magnetic stimulation
26. ToM - Theory of Mind
27. TRENDS - Tool for Recognition of Emotions in Neuropsychiatric Disorders
28. WL - Waitlist
29. YT - Yoga therapy

# ABSTRACT

## INTRODUCTION

Schizophrenia is a severe mental disorder affecting young adults with a lifetime prevalence of 1%. It's characterized by three important symptom clusters namely positive, negative & cognitive symptoms. Except for the positive symptoms, there are no effective treatments available for the negative and cognitive symptoms. In addition, the existing treatments are not free of side effects; some causing extrapyramidal side effects and others causing metabolic side effects.

Unavailability of effective biological treatments for negative and cognitive symptoms adds to the already existing burden of socio-occupational dysfunction associated with these symptom clusters. Psychosocial interventions are available targeting a few or most of the domains of social cognition with or without neurocognition training. But majority of them [for example, Cognitive Enhancement Therapy(CET), Social Cognition Interaction Training(SCIT)] are highly resource intensive and its feasibility in developing countries are questionable, though they might be effective. Moreover, they were developed among the western patient population and its cultural validity in eastern countries with more of religious inclination is yet to be tested. Hence, there is a need to explore the role of other complementary therapies like yoga for an integrated approach in treating patients with schizophrenia.

Yoga as a mind-body therapy is useful in lifestyle related disorders, including neuropsychiatric disorders. In healthy adults and elderly, yoga is found to be efficacious in improving cognitive skills. Yoga has been shown to significantly improve negative symptoms and functioning in schizophrenia patients. In a recent study, along with improvements in functioning, yoga also increased oxytocin levels along with improvement in Facial Emotion Recognition Deficit (FERD) in patients with schizophrenia.(Jayaram et al., 2013). In this study, we hypothesized that practice of yoga for one month would improve social cognition in patients with schizophrenia.

## LITERARY REVIEW

Yoga being a science of spirituality, does not have direct descriptions related to any disorder including schizophrenia. Hence Ayurveda -one of the ancient literatures on health and disorders, is focused elaboratively pertaining to psychosis and its management with a brief review on mind, different states of mind & control of mind as per *Yoga vāsiśṭha, Māṇḍūkya Upaniṣad, Shiva Swarodaya, Hatha Yoga Pradipika and Patanjali Yoga Sutra.* Concepts of social cognition described in yoga literatures has been explored.

In the modern scientific literature, with a brief outline on social cognition, all the available psychosocial interventions for social cognition improvement has been reviewed thoroughly and the need for complementary therapies like yoga for social cognitive deficits in schizophrenia is emphasized.

## AIM

To study the effect of yoga-based intervention on social cognition in patients with schizophrenia.

## OBJECTIVES

Primary:

1. To study the effect of add-on yoga therapy on Social Cognition measures (composite score of SOCRATIS and TRENDS)

Secondary:

1. To study the effect of add-on yoga therapy on Mirror Neuron Activity (MNA) using functional Near Infrared Spectroscopy (fNIRS) in patients with schizophrenia

## METHODS

Study was conducted at National Institute of Mental Health & Neurosciences (NIMHANS) at Bengaluru in collaboration with S-VYASA Yoga University. Study design was Randomized Controlled Trial (RCT)

Schizophrenia patients attending services at psychiatry department (outpatients=29; inpatients=11) of NIMHANS, were assessed for eligibility by a psychiatry resident and the diagnosis was confirmed using Mini-International

Neuro Psychiatric Interview (MINI). With written informed consent, patients who were stabilized on antipsychotics for at least 6 weeks and were co-operative for yoga practices were recruited. The data was collected from March 2016 to July 2017. Random assignment of eligible and willing subjects to Yoga Therapy Group(YT) or Waitlist Control (WL) was done by the research scholar with Sequentially Numbered Opaque Sealed Envelope(SNOSE) method. Computer generated random numbers were used for treatment assignment. Random numbers were generated by a scientific officer who was not involved in assessment or recruitment of the subjects.

The subjects recruited were of either gender, coming from the age group of 18-45 years with Clinical Global Impression-Severity(CGI-S)(Guy W, 2000) score of 3 or more. Patients with history of risk of harm to self or others; who had received Electroconvulsive Therapy (ECT) or Yoga therapy in the last six months; patients with significant neurological disorder or head injury; patients with substance abuse in last one month or dependence in last six months except nicotine were excluded.

Validated Yoga module was administered to the Yoga group for 60 min, 4-5 sessions per week, with a total of 20 sessions to be completed within 6 weeks. Maximum 3 subjects were taught together in a session. Waitlist participants were offered Yoga after 6 weeks.

All the subjects underwent the following assessments,

1) Social Cognition Rating Tool in Indian Setting (SOCRATIS)
2) Scale for Assessment of Negative Symptoms (SANS)
3) Scale for Assessment of Positive Symptoms (SAPS)
4) Groningen Social Disabilities Schedule (GSDS-II)
5) Clinical Global Impression (CGI)
6) Brief Cognitive Assessment Tool for Schizophrenia (B-CATS) comprising of three tasks i.e., Digit Symbol-Coding, Semantic Fluency, and Trail Making Test-B
7) Mirror Neuron Activity (MNA) assessment by functional Near Infrared Spectroscopy (fNIRS)

A trained yoga therapist gave the yoga intervention to subjects. A Psychiatry resident did the clinical assessments and was blind to the treatment allocation. Clinical assessments (positive symptoms, negative symptoms and social disability/functioning) which are subjective were assessed by a blind assessor (Psychiatry resident) and the social cognition assessment which is a computer based objective test (less prone to bias), was done by non-blinded research scholar.

## RESULTS

Out of 478 screened subjects, 339 were eligible for study and 40 eligible subjects agreed for participation in the study.

Data was analyzed with SPSS (version 24). Data was screened for outliers and tested for normality. Baseline and demographic data for the groups were comparable.

The results can be summarized as follows,

After 6 weeks of add-on yoga therapy, there was significant improvement over time and between the groups favoring yoga intervention for Social Cognition Composite Score (SCCS), SANS & GSDS; there was significant improvement over time but not between groups for SAPS and Verbal Fluency Test (VFT); Digit Symbol Substitution Test (DSST) and Colour Trial-B (CT) neither showed significant change over time nor between groups.

There was no Mirror Neuron Activity(MNA) at Left Ventral Premotor Cortex, measured by fNIRS. Hence further comparison of MNA between pre- and post-intervention and between groups was not done.

## DISCUSSION

Social cognition & MNA:

This is one of the first studies exploring the role of yoga in social cognition. Previous studies have looked into the effect of yoga on Facial Emotion Recognition Deficit (FERD) in patients with schizophrenia. Previous studies (Jayaram et al., 2013) (R V Behere et al., 2011) have shown that yoga improves FERD in patients with schizophrenia. In this current study, social cognition is measured as a composite score which includes ToM (1st order and 2nd order), FERD, Social perception and Attribution Style (AS).

In our study, failure to detect the presence of MNA could be due to inadequate sample size. This is one of the first studies using fNIRS to assess MNA the possibility of studying MNA with fNIRS and hence its utility with yoga intervention needs to be tested with adequate sample size.

Clinical symptoms & Social functioning:

Results of this study is consistent with previous studies (Duraiswamy, Thirthalli, Nagendra, & Gangadhar, 2007) (Varambally et al., 2012) (Jayaram et al., 2013) (R V Behere et al., 2011) which shows that yoga is useful in improving negative symptoms (measured by SANS) more than the positive symptoms (measured by SAPS). Improvement in the social functioning along with the negative symptoms following yoga suggest that these may be related to each other as evidenced by prior studies.

Neuropsychological tests:

There was no significant improvement in any of the neuropsychological tests scores (VFT, DSST, CT-B) following yoga intervention. Previous studies with yoga intervention were mainly on healthy population. One of the consistent findings in majority of prior studies were improvement in attention (Gothe & McAuley, 2015)

Yoga could possibly work by both bottom-up and top-down approaches - promoting relaxation through asana and pranayama, and mindfulness through chanting and positive resolution respectively. This dual effect of Yoga might well fit in with the dual processing theory of Social Cognition (Evans, 2008) , with mindfulness (yoga mediated) promoting controlled (reflective) processing and relaxation modulating the reflexive (automatic) processing.

## CONCLUSION

One-month add-on yoga therapy improves social cognition, negative symptoms and social functioning. Add-on yoga therapy could also be considered along with available social cognition interventions, especially in Indian setup, as it is more culturally acceptable and feasible for its applications in clinical setup.

## CONTENTS

## LIST OF TABLES

## LIST OF FIGURES

# Chapter 1.0
# INTRODUCTION

# 1.0 INTRODUCTION

Schizophrenia is a chronic psychotic disorder affecting 1% of world population. The three important symptom clusters in schizophrenia are as follows,

Positive symptoms (Hallucinations, Delusions, Disorganization), Negative symptoms (Avolition, Apathy, Alogia, Asociality, Affective flattening) and Cognitive symptoms (Attention, Executive function, Working memory & Episodic memory impairment and social cognition impairment).

As conceptualized by Kraepelin, cognitive impairment is very much central to schizophrenia. It begins early in the course of schizophrenia and persist even after the remission of other symptoms. It's also related to the negative symptoms and social-occupational functioning.

Cognitive deficit in schizophrenia covers both neuro cognition and social cognition. Neurocognitive deficits are more pronounced in attention, working memory, problem solving, processing speed(Steven D, Targum MD and Richard S.E. Keefe, 2008). Many targeted treatment approaches like cognitive remediation therapy are available for improving neurocognitive deficit. Though social cognition deficit is strongly correlated with functional outcome, it has not been the focus for many decades, as it was understood as a subset of neurocognition.

But recent evidences suggest that social cognition is not just neurocognition applied in social situations. Though overlapping, social cognition is distinct from neurocognition in many aspects including its independent neural pathways and its strong impact on functional outcome(Fett, Viechtbauer, Penn, van Os, & Krabbendam, 2011). Considering the significance of social cognition, NIMH-MATRICS (National Institute of Mental Health- Measurement and Treatment Research to Improve Cognition in Schizophrenia) initiative had considered social cognition in schizophrenia as a central topic and included it as one of the seven domains in the MATRICS consensus cognitive battery for clinical trials in schizophrenia.

In the recent years, there has been increased number of publications exponentially, in the area of social cognition in schizophrenia (Fig-1.1). It has led to development of many treatment approaches for enhancing the social cognitive deficit in schizophrenia, majority of them being psychosocial interventions few being pharmacological interventions.

In spite of availability of varied modern medical interventions, increased disability in terms of social and functional outcome is still a major concern. Because atypical antipsychotics which are the main stay of treatment in schizophrenia, do not help much in management of cognitive symptoms and negative symptoms(Szöke, Trandafir, Dupont, Méary, Schürhoff, & Leboyer, 2008)(Joanna Moncrieff, 2011). In fact, the functional outcome in terms of a productive life, economically and socially,

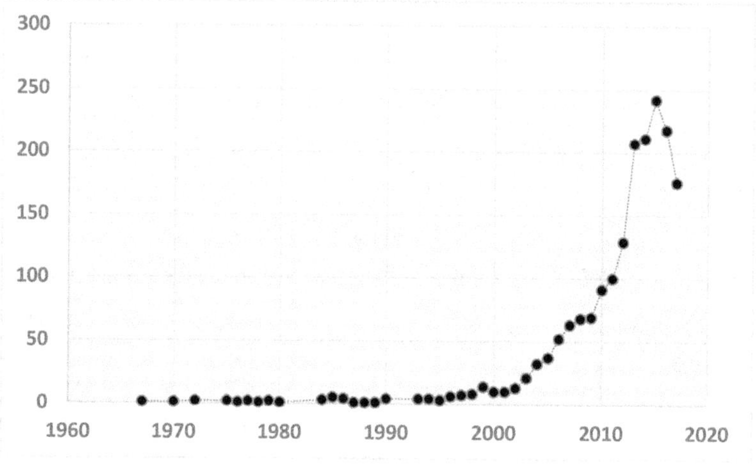


**Figure – 1.1 Social cognition research in schizophrenia**

which is very much related to the cognitive function is severely impaired and constitutes the major cost burden of schizophrenia.

On the other hand, psychosocial interventions like Cognitive Enhancement Therapy(CET), Social Cognition Interaction Training (SCIT) are very much resource intensive. Moreover, these psychosocial interventions developed in western countries were found to be efficacious in their patient population. Its cultural validity for eastern countries like India is yet to be investigated.

Adding to this deadlock in the treatment of cognitive symptoms (including social cognitive deficit) is the complexity of the concept of social cognition itself. Until the recent NIMH workshop in 2006 at USA, social cognition and its domains were not clear for the researchers in schizophrenia patient population. The workshop consensus statement has given guidelines on various domains of social cognition (Theory of Mind, Emotion processing, Attribution style, Social perception and social knowledge) for its utility in research in schizophrenia. However, these guidelines were only a beginning to explore and understand the social cognitive deficit in schizophrenia.

A recent review by Green et al, clarifies the evolving and dynamic nature of social cognition including and hence the complexity of investigating the social cognition especially in schizophrenia patient population. This review tried to conceptualize the concept of social cognition in a broader, social psychological perspective by clubbing all the social cognitive impairments under two categories-impairment in reflective processing and reflexive processing. Summary of the review is shown in fig-1.2. This dual processing theory of reflective and reflexive processing would fit well with the of hypo frontality and dopamine salience hypothesis of schizophrenia.

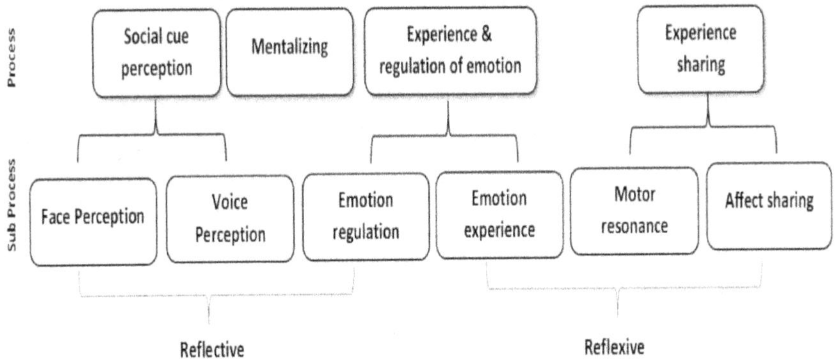


**Fig-1.2 Social cognition process & sub process (from Green et al, 2015)**

So, on one hand, concept of social cognition and the underlying mechanisms are being evolved and on the other hand, social cognitive interventions are simultaneously developed targeting a particular domain of social cognition or on a broad-based approach.

In this context of evolving concepts/mechanisms and intervention for social cognition in schizophrenia, our study had two broad aims,

1) To investigate the effect of add-on yoga therapy on social cognition in schizophrenia

2) To explore the possible connection between Mirror Neuron Activity (MNA) measured by functional Near Infra Red Spectroscopy (fNIRS) and social cognition including the clinical and functional outcomes in schizophrenia.

Studying the role of add-on yoga therapy intervention is relevant, considering the resource intensiveness of available psychosocial interventions; cultural diversity of social cognition aspects (most of the available psychosocial interventions are developed in western population) and easy acceptability of yoga based interventions in Eastern countries like India. Previous studies with yoga intervention have shown to improve clinical symptoms, functional outcome and some aspects of social cognition like Facial Emotion Recognition and plasma oxytocin levels in patients with schizophrenia. Hence the current study focused on all the four domains of social cognition measured by SOCRATIS (Social Cognition Rating Tool for Indian Setup)-Theory of Mind (ToM), Attribution style, social perception and Emotion processing assessed by TRENDS (Tool for Recognizing Emotions in Neuropsychiatric DisorderS).

We have also aimed at exploring the relation between MNA and clinical symptoms including social cognition as it would enhance the scientific knowledge for refining the social cognition interventions in the future for the betterment of the patient population.

In our study, MNA was studied with fNIRS unlike previous studies which has used fMRI (functional Magnetic Resonance Imaging), TMS (Transcranial Magnetic Stimulation), EEG (Electroencephalograph) & MEG (Magnetic Encephalograph) (indirect measurements) or direct single cell recording. fNIRS works on the principle of neurovascular coupling similar to fMRI. Using fNIRS is unique in two ways,

1) Cost effective compared to all the other modalities

2) Motor paradigms could be used for eliciting MNA, without any motion artefacts unlike other imaging modalities.

In our study, we used fNIRS with conventional MNA paradigms (observing a pincer hand grasp video and static image). Along with the conventional paradigms, we also used a motor task paradigm (subject performing a motor task while undergoing fNIRS recording) for eliciting MNA.

# Chapter 2.0
# LITERARY RESEARCH

# 2.0 LITERARY RESEARCH

Yoga being a science of spirituality, does not have direct descriptions related to any disorder including schizophrenia. Hence Ayurveda -one of the ancient literatures on health and disorders, is focused elaboratively pertaining to psychosis and its management with a brief review on mind, different states of mind & control of mind as per *Yoga vāsiśṭha, Māṇḍūkya Upaniṣad, Shiva Swarodaya, Hatha Yoga Pradipika and Patanjali Yoga Sutra.*

## 2.1 MIND ACCORDING TO YOGIC SCRIPTURES

***Concept of mind:***

Concept of mind in yogic scriptures is different compared to modern psychology.

According to yoga literature, mind has four aspects*(antaḥkaraṇa)* namely,

*manas*(mind),
*buddhi* (intellect),
*ahaṅkāra* (ego)
*citta* (memory)
*manas* is the conglomeration of thoughts, *buddhi* is that which decides or discriminates, *ahaṅkāra* is the sense of 'I'ness and *citta* is the collection of experiences cognitive and emotional.

---

*saṁkalpavikalpātakaṁ manaḥ*|
*niścayātmikā buddhiḥ*|
*āhaṁkartā ahaṅkāraḥ cintanakartṛ cittam*|
*Tattvabodha, Ch: 35, V:1*

---

***States of mind:***

Sage Vyasa's commentary to *Patanjali Yoga Sutra* defines five states of mind as follows,

*kṣipta* (disturbed), *mūḍha* (dull), *vikṣipta* (distracted), *ekāgra* (one pointed) and *niruddha* (mastered)

*Kṣipta*

This state is fully dominated by the guna *'rajas'*. In this state, the mind is totally restless, jumping from one thought to another, from one emotion to the next and from object to the next.

*Mūḍha*

The *mūḍha* state is dominated by the guna 'tamas' in which the mind is dull, sleepy, lethargic and lacking any alertness. In the *mūḍha* state no productive work can be achieved.

*Vikṣipta*

There are moments when the sattva *guna* begins to dominate and the mind can find moments of focus and concentration. However, old habits keep pulling the mind away from sattva and back to rajas or tamas. The vikṣipta state represents this pulling away from the partial state of concentration.

*Ekāgra*

In this state the mind is fully focused on the object of meditation and the object becomes fully illuminated, realized and completely known.

*Niruddha*

In this state no new *samskaras* (impressions) can arise. Even though past impressions still remain, they are made ineffective and can no longer cause any afflictions. In the state of *niruddha* the mind continues to provide its normal functionality. However, it is now fully under the control of the yogi and all the vrittis (fluctuations) that happen are under the control of the pure, *sattvic buddhi* (intellect) as opposed to being controlled by the ego.

*kṣiptaṁ mūḍhaṁ vikṣiptaṁ ekāgraṁ niruddham iti cittabhūmayaḥ*

*Yoga vāsiṣṭha* also explains about wavering mind as follows,

*cetaścañcalayā vṛttyā cintānicayacañcuram|*
*ḍhṛtiṁ badhnāti naikatra pañjare kesari yathā|*

*cetaḥ patati kāryeṣu vigataḥ svāmiṣeṣviva|*
*kṣṇena viranti yāti bālaḥ krīḍana kādiva||*
*Yoga vāsiṣṭha Ch: I, V: 5 & 6*

---

***Controlling the mind:***

In yogic tradition, mind is controlled by using an object of focus. The object could be external or internal. Breath is one of the important tool used for controlling the mind. The practice of focusing the mind on object of concentration is spiritually called as d*hāraṇā.*

*Dhāraṇā* as a tool:

*Dhāraṇā is* the sixth limb in *Patanjali's ashtang yoga*. It is focusing the mind on an object of concentration

---

*deśa-bandhaḥ cittasya dhāraṇā.*
*PSY Ch: III, V:1*

---

Sage Vyasa further explains about different objects for concentration as follows,

---

*ṇābhicakre hṛdayapuṇḍarīke mūrdhni jyotiṣi nāsikāgre jihvāgre ityevamādiṣu deśeṣu bāhye vā viṣaye cittasya vṛttimātreṇa bandha iti dhāraṇā|1|*

Dharana is fixing the mind, through its modifications, to places such as the navel circle, the heart lotus, the shining centre in the head, the tip of the nose, the tip of the tongue, and other such locations; and to external objects.

Another important technique of controlling the mind according to *Māṇḍūkya Upaniṣad* is, activating the mind when it is dull and quietening the mind when it is agitated. The equanimity that would be experienced by this practice, has to be enhanced gradually until it becomes natural. The verse which explain this technique is as follows,

*laye sambodhayet cittaṁ vikṣiptaṁ śamayet punaḥ*
*sakaṣāyaṁ vijñānīyāt samaprāptaṁ na cālayet|*
*Māṇḍūkya Upaniṣad kārikā:* 3.44

'In a state of mental inactivity awaken the mind; when agitated, calm it; between these two states realize the possible abilities of the mind. If the mind has reached the state of perfect equilibrium then do not disturb it again'

Breath as a tool (for *dhāraṇā.*):

Amongst the various objects of focus used for *dhāraṇā,* breath is the most commonly and easily used tool. The relation between breath flow and cerebral activity/laterality is well explained in

1) Swara yoga text- Shiva Swarodaya

2) Hatha yoga scriptures

*1) Swara yoga* on cerebral dominance/laterality:

"Swara" etymologically means the sound of one's own breath. Swara yoga emphasizes the analysis of breath flow and utilizing the knowledge for modifying the cerebral activity.

Swara yoga explains that the two-major energy*(prana*) circuits, *ida* and *pingala*, can be regulated and controlled by means of the breath.

According to swara yoga ida, the negative channel, emanates and terminates on the left side, and has greater control over the left half of the body. Conversely, pingala, the positive channel, emanates and terminates on the right side and its influence is greater on the right half of the body. So, if there is disturbance in the rhythm or cycles of the breath, there is likely to be some imbalance in the whole-body system including the cerebral hemispheres.

*Ida* corresponds to flow of breath in the left nostril (impacting the right cerebral hemisphere) and *pingala* corresponds to flow of breath in right nostril (impacting the left cerebral hemisphere). This relationship of breath flow in the nostril with the corresponding cerebral laterality has been demonstrated with EEG recordings (Werntz, Bickford, Bloom, & Shannahoff-Khalsa, 1982)

---

*iḍā vāme sthitā bhāge pingalā dakśiṇe smrutā|* 38

*Shiva Swarodaya Verse:8*

---

This knowledge of swara yoga is important for two reasons

a) Breath can be manipulated to alter the cerebral activity

b) Breath manipulation for modifying the cerebral activity could be used in schizophrenia, which is conceived as a disorder of left hemisphere dysfunction (ref sommer 2001)

2) Hatha yoga on *Kaphalbhati*

The word "kaphal" means skull and "bhati" means shining or illuminating. Kaphalbhati is a high frequency breathing which removes excess kapha and the frontal brain.

*bhastrāvalloha-kārasya recha-pūrau sasambhramau |*

*kapālabhātirvikhyātā kapha-doṣha-viśoṣhaṇī || 35 ||*

*Hatha Yoga Pradipika Ch-2; V:35*

Similar to Kaphalbhati is the practice of Bhastrika, which activates the whole brain rather than the frontal brain.

Practices like Kaphalbhati & Bhastrika, (which activates the frontal/whole brain) are important in the context of schizophrenia, as it is established that frontal dysfunction is one of the key features of schizophrenia.

## 2.2 SCHIZOPHRENIA ACCORDING TO AYURVEDA:

Psychosis and related symptoms are described under the name of *unmāda* in *charak saṁhitā.* The term *unmāda* stands for *samudbhrama* i.e perversion.

*Unmāda* is characterized by perversion of mind, intellect, consciousness, knowledge, memory, desires, manners, behaviours and interaction with others.

*samudbhramaṁ buddhimanaḥ smṛtīnāmunmādamagantunijotthamāhuḥ|8|*

*Caraka-saṃhitā, Cikitsā sthāna Ch:9 V:8*

It's postulated that imbalances in the *doṣā* leads to diseases in general including *unmāda.*

**Etiology of *unmāda:***

1) Intake of v*iruddha* (mutually contradictory), *dushta* (polluted) and *ashuchi* (impure) foods and drinks

2) *Pradharsana* (insult) to the Gods, Gurus and elders.

3) Affliction of the mind because of fear and sudden happiness

4) Unwholesome physical and mental activities

---

*viruddha duṣṭāśuci bhojanāni pradharṣaṇaṁ deva guru dvijānām|*

*unmāda heturbhaya harṣa pūrvo manobhighāto viṣamāśca ceṣṭāḥ|4|*

*Caraka-saṃhitā, Cikitsā sthāna Ch:9 V:4*

---

***Pathogenesis of unmāda:***

Vitiation of *doṣā* affects the *hrudaya* (the abode of intellect) of a person having less of *sattva*. It also afflicts the channels carrying psychic impulse and hence the mind.

---

*tairalpa sattvasya malāḥ praduṣḥā buddhernivāsaṁ hṛdayaṁ pradūṣya|*

*srotāsyadhiṣṭhāya manovahāni pramohayantyāśu narasya cetaḥ||5||*

*Caraka-saṃhitā, Cikitsā sthāna Ch:9 V:5*

---

***General signs & symptoms:***

Some of the common symptoms are intellectual confusion, fickleness of mind, impatience, irrelevant speech and a sensation of vacuum in the heart (empty mindedness) *dhī vibhramaḥ sattva pariplavaśca paryākulā dṛṣṭiradhīratā ca|*

*abaddhavāktvaṁ hṛdayaṁ ca śūnyaṁ sāmānyamunmādagadasya liṅgam||6||*

*sa mūḍhacetā na sukhaṁ na duḥkhaṁ nācāradharmau kuta eva śāntim|*

*vindatyapāstasmṛtibuddhisajo bhramatyayaṁ ceta itastataśca||7||*

*Caraka-saṃhitā, Cikitsā sthāna Ch:9 V:6 & 7*

***Types of unmāda***

*Unmāda* could be due to endogenous or exogenous cause. *Unmāda* due to imbalance in the *doṣā* is classified as endogenous *unmāda* and exogenous type includes *unmāda* caused by etiological factors other than vitiation of *doṣā*

Endogenous type includes *vataja unmāda, paittika unmāda, slaismika unmāda, sannipatika unmāda.*

*Vataja unmāda*

Characterized by an emaciated body, inappropriate lamenting, shouting, laughing, dancing, singing, playing music, posturing; repeatedly and tunelessly imitating the sound of a flute, veena, or other instrument; frothing at the mouth; constantly wandering about; ceaseless talking; using things which are not ornaments as decoration; trying to travel on things which are not vehicles; being greedy for food, but spurning it once it has been obtained.

*rūkṣālpa śītānna vireka dhātu kṣayopavāsairanilotivṛddhaḥ|*

*cintādi juṣṭaṁ hṛdayaṁ pradūṣya buddhiṁ smṛtiṁ cāpyupahanti śīghram||*

*9|| asthānahāsasmitanṛtyagītavāgaṅgavikṣepaṇarodanāni|*

*pāruṣya kārśyāruṇa varṇatāśca jīrṇe balaṁ cānilajasya rūpam||10||*

*Caraka-saṃhitā, Cikitsā sthāna Ch:9 V:9 & 10*

---

*Pittaja unmāda*

Characterized by threatening behavior & charging at people with stones inappropriately. The patient craves cool shade, water, goes naked, and has a yellow color. He/she sees thing which are not there, such as fire, flames, stars, and lamps. Pittaja insanity results from indigestion, excess of hot, pungent, sour, or burning foods and liquids

---

*ajīrṇa kaṭvamla vidāhyaśītairbhojyaiścitaṁ pittamudīrṇavegam|*

*unmādamatyugramanātmakasya hṛdi śritaṁ pūrvavadāśu kuryāt||*

*11|| amarṣa saṁrambha vinagnabhāvāḥ*

*santarjanātidravaṇauṣṇyaroṣāḥ | praccāyaśītānnajalābhilāṣaḥ pītā*

*ca bhāḥ pittakṛtasya liṅgam||12||*

*Caraka-saṃhitā, Cikitsā sthāna Ch:9 V:11 & 12*

*Kaphaja unmāda*

Characterized by vomiting and a reduction in motivation, appetite, and conversation. It causes a lust for women. It causes the patient to enjoy solitude. He/she dribbles mucus and is very frightening; hates being clean. This *unmāda* is stronger at night, and just after eating.

*sampūraṇairmanda viceṣṭitasya soṣmā kapho marmaṇi sampravṛddhaḥ|*

*buddhiṁ smṛtiṁ cāpyupahatya cittaṁ pramohayan sajanayedvikāram||13||*

*vākceṣṭitaṁ mandamarocakaśca nārīviviktapriyatātinidrā|*

*cardiśca lālā ca balaṁ ca bhuṅkte nakhādiśauklyaṁ ca kaphātmakasya||14||*

*Caraka-saṃhitā, Cikitsā sthāna Ch:9 V:13 & 14*

*Sannipatika unmāda*

Characterized by all the above-mentioned symptoms simultaneously. It's considered to be incurable.

*yaḥ sannipāta prabhavotighoraḥ sarvaiḥ samastaiḥ sa ca hetubhiḥ syāt|*

*sarvāṇi rūpāṇi bibharti tādṛgvirudghabhaiṣajyavidhirvivarjyaḥ||15||*

*Caraka-saṃhitā, Cikitsā sthāna Ch:9 V:15*

---

Exogenous *unmāda (Agantuja unmāda)*

Exogenous type of *unmāda* is caused by improper observance of *niyama* (spiritual disciplines) in the present life and improper conduct of the past life which leads to seizures by the Gods, Rishis (Sages), Rakshas (demons) and Pitrus (ancestors)

---

*devarṣi gandharva piśāca yakṣa rakṣaḥpitṛiṇāmabhidharṣaṇāni|*

*āgantu heturniyamavratādi mithyākṛtaṁ karma ca pūrvadehe||16||*

*Caraka-saṃhitā, Cikitsā sthāna Ch:9 V:16*

---

Scholars believe that the *Agantuja unmāda* is caused by one's own sinful activities. Some believe it to be caused by intellectual blasphemy. Patient disregards the Gods, ascetics, ancestors, teachers and the other respectable ones. They also resort to undesirable inauspicious activities leading to insanity.

Subtypes of exogenous *unmāda:*

*Devonmāda:*

The patient would have a gentle look, free from anger, sleep and desire for food, having less of sweat, urine, stool and flatus. He/She emits good aroma from the body and face may look like a blooming lotus.

Guru *unmāda :*

These patients would have activities and speech as ordained by their preceptors.

*Pitru unmāda:*

This type of patients would look drowsy with interrupted speech and lack of desire for food.

Gandharva *unmāda:*

Characterised by violent acts, seriousness, invincibility and liking for dancing, singing, good food, good drinks, incense, perfume, laughing and talking (engagement in humorous talks). Pleasuring aroma would come out from their body.

*Yakshonmāda* :

Characterized by frequent sleep, cry and laugh, liking for dancing, singing, playing musical instruments, reciting sacred scriptures, telling stories, good food, drinks, bath, garlands, incense and perfumes. Eyes would be red and tearful. Patient would talk ill of elders and may disclose the secrets of others.

*Rakshasonmāda*:

Characterized by sleeplessness, hatred for food and drinks, excessive strength of patient in spite of his aversion for food, liking for weapons, blood, meat and red garlands and ferociousness.

*Brahma Rakshasa unmāda:*

Characterized by excessive laughter, dance, hatred and disobedience to the Gods, Vipras (persons belonging to the family of Brahmins) and Physicians. May be proficient in reciting hymns from the Vedas and other scriptures. They might harm themselves.

*Pishachonmāda*:

Characterized by fickle mindedness. May engage themselves in dancing, singing, laughing and incoherent speech. They may like climbing over uneven places, entering into caves, walking in dirty streets and over dirty clothes, and climbing over heaps of grass, stones and woods. Voice would be broken and hoarse. May remain naked and run here and there. They won't stick to one place.

***Management of unmāda:***

1. *Snehapana* (internal oleation with medicated ghee)
2. *Mridu shodhana* (mild body purification by emesis or purgation)
3. *Niruha basti* (decoction enema)
4. *Shirovirechana* (medicated nasal drops) and
5. *Sanjna prabodhana* (oral medication to stabilize the mind)

Formulations recommended in *unmāda*:

*1. Kalyanaka ghrita*

*2. Mahakalyanaka ghrita*

*3. Mahapaishacha ghrita*

*4. Lashunadya ghrita*

*4. Unmade gajanakusha rasa*

*6. Saraswata choorna*

*7. Sarsawatarishta*

*8. Sarpagandha ghanavati*

*9. Brihatvata chintamani*

*10. Yogendra rasa*

Specific management guidelines as per the type of *unmāda:*

In *vataja unmāda*, the physician should first of all ascertain the nature of *vata*, and in the beginning, administer Sneha (oil, Ghee, etc). If the passage of *vata* is obstructed, then the patient is given laxative along with Sneha (oil, ghee etc) only in small quantities.

If caused by *kapha or pitta*, *vamana and virechana* treatments are given, after *snehana* and *swedana*. These therapies are followed up with *samsarjana Krama* (from lighter to heavier diet gradually).

Thereafter, he is given *niruha* (decoction enema), *sneha basti* (oil / fat enema) and *nasya* therapy (therapies for the elimination of *dosha* from the head). Depending upon the predominance of *dosha*, these elimination therapies are required to be administered repeatedly *unmāde vātaje pūrvaṁ snehapānaṁ viśeṣavit|*

*kuryādāvṛtamārge tu sasnehaṁ mṛdu śodhanam||25||*

*kaphapittodbhavepyādau vamanaṁ savirecanam|*

*snigdhasvinnasya kartavyaṁ śuddhe saṁsarjanakramaḥ||26||*

*nirūhaṁ snehabastiṁ ca śirasaśca virecanam|*

*tataḥ kuryādyathādoṣaṁ teṣāṁ bhūyastvamācaret||27||*

*hṛdindriyaśiraḥkoṣṭhe saṁśuddhe vamanādibhiḥ|*

*manaḥprasādamāpnoti smṛtiṁ sajāṁ ca vindati||28||*

*śuddhasyācāravibhraṁśe tīkṣṇaṁ nāvanamajanam| tāḍanaṁ*

*ca manobuddhidehasaṁvejanaṁ hitam||29||*

*yaḥ saktovinaye paṭṭaiḥ saṁyamya sudṛḍhaiḥ sukhaiḥ|*

*apetalohakāṣṭhādye saṁrodhyaśca tamogṛhe||30||*

*tarjanaṁ trāsanaṁ dānaṁ harṣaṇaṁ sāntvanaṁ bhayam|*

*vismayo vismṛterhetornayanti prakṛtiṁ manaḥ||31||*

*pradehotsādanābhyaṅgadhūmāḥ pānaṁ ca sarpiṣaḥ|*

*prayoktavyaṁ manobuddhismṛtisajāprabodhanam||32||*

*sarpiḥpānādirāgantormantrādiścesyate vidhiḥ|33|*

*Caraka-saṃhitā, Cikitsā sthāna Ch:9 V:25-33*

---

***Use of panchakarma treatment:***

By the administration of *vamana* therapies, the heart, sense organs, head and koshta (Gastro- intestinal tract) gets cleaned as a result of which, the mind gets refreshed and the patient gains memory as well as consciousness. If, even after the body is cleansed, the patient exhibits perversion of conduct, then he is given *teekhsna navana nasya* – strong inhalation therapy.

*Teekshna Anjana* – collieries and even beatings which are useful for stimulating his mind, intellect and the body are tried. If the patient has a strong physique, and he/she is disobedient, then he/she is tied tightly without hurting his body, with pieces of cloth, and kept confined to a dark room devoid of iron (rods) and wooden pieces.

The patient suffering from *Agantuja unmāda* is given p*ana* (to be taken internally) and mantras to be recited for betterment.

## 2.3 CONCEPT OF COGNITION IN THE CONTEXT OF YOGA

Cognition is defined as the mental process of acquiring knowledge and understanding through thought, experience and the senses.

According to Patanjali, knowledge can be acquired by direct perception through senses, inference, scriptural references or from person who is authority on scriptures (Iyengar BKS, 2007)

Examples:

Direct perception through senses: feeling cold in a winter season

Inferential knowledge: Inferring the possibility of fire by seeing smoke on a hill top

Scriptures/Person of Wisdom: Desire is the root cause of all our problems

***Understanding Social Cognition in the context of Yoga:***

Social cognition is defined as mental operations underlying social interactions(Brothers, 1990).

In psychological terms, attribution forms the core of this mental operations guiding our social behaviour. Attribution is the ability to understand and attribute causality for any event happening in our surroundings. Attributing cause could be based on facts, sense perception, past experience or based on one's belief system. For example, Mr A might feel "he (Mr B) looks very sad and depressed" so let me do prayer for him. Now this single thought would guide the whole set of interactions which Mr A might have with Mr B. Mr A attributes the cause for sadness to something unknown and he believes prayer would help him. If Mr A feels Mr B is a wicked person, then there is chance Mr A might attribute the sadness for Mr B's misdeeds also and his behaviour might vary accordingly. So everything is hinged on how do we understand our self (beliefs, intentions, etc..) and others (their beliefs, intentions, etc..)

Attribution is based on one's beliefs, intentions and also how one perceives the same in other's too. Interestingly sage Patanjali discusses similar concept as *anumāna* (one of the tool for acquiring knowledge. Example-Inferring possibility of fire, on seeing smoke over a hill top)). This tool of inference (*anumāna*) would apply very well to the context of social interactions as well. This concept of *anumāna* described by Patanjali is strikingly similar to the concept of Theory of Mind (ToM) popular in the field of social cognition. As the name suggest, it's theorizing about one's mind, which may or may not be correct, but is very essential for social interaction. The very term *anumāna (anumāna* means suspecting/guessing) also means theorizing possible causes for an event (Example- "he is crying because, somebody would have scolded him". "Somebody would have scolded" is just a guess/suspicion/theory, it may or may not be true). Though Yoga is a text developed for the inner growth of spiritual aspirant, it does have concepts of social cognition applicable in a therapeutic context as well, which could be used with appropriate modifications in therapy.

Interestingly, Patanjali who defines yoga as *citta-vṛtti-nirodhaḥ* (PYS: I-2) (cessation of *vṛtti* is yoga), mentions knowledge (attained by any of these means) also, as one of the sources of vrittis. Illusion, delusion, sleep and memory are other sources of *vṛtti* (PYS: I-6). Possibly Patanjali agrees that at an ordinary level, all the tools of acquiring knowledge are not entirely fool proof, as until one gets perfection (mostly an ideal concept, not practical in today's world) all the inferences and hence the social or non-social interactions would be coloured by one's own beliefs and intentions which are inherent in all our decisions and inferences.

Recognizing this notion that understanding oneself (including beliefs, desires and intentions) plays a pivotal role in all our interactions with the self and others (similar to simulation theory of ToM), Patanjali says in the third verse of first chapter, "a seer dwells in his original state" (PYS:I-3) (*svarūpa* -pure consciousness which is not coloured by beliefs and intentions) so that the perception, attribution and ensuing interactions (social/non-social) would be least distorted by one's own beliefs and attitudes.

Going beyond the level of an ordinary person, Patanjali describes a higher level of social connection similar to extra sensory perceptions for aspirants who can focus on the nature of one's pure-self more intensely.

Some of the experiences which Patanjali discusses are

By *samyama*, one gains the knowledge of the language of all beings (PYS: III-19); acquires the ability to understand the minds of others, divine faculties of hearing, touch, vision, taste and smell (PYS: III-37)

Selected Verses from Patanjali Yoga Sutras (PYS)

---

*yogaś-citta-vṛtti-nirodhaḥ ||PYS: I-2||*

*tadā draṣṭuḥ svarūpe-'vasthānam ||PYS: I-3||*

*pramāṇa viparyaya vikalpa nidrā smṛtayaḥ ||PYS: I-6||*

*pratyakṣa-anumāna-āgamāḥ pramāṇāni ||PYS: I-7||*

*pratyayasya para-citta-jñānam* ||*PYS: III-19*||

*te samādhav-upasargā[ḥ]-vyutthāne siddhayaḥ* ||*PYS: III-37*||

## 2.4 SUMMARY OF TRADITIONAL LITERATURE REVIEW

Ayurveda has its own classification of *unmāda*- a concept similar to psychosis. Broadly classified as endogenous and exogenous *unmāda.* Specific treatments are also prescribed depending on the type of *unmāda.*

Concepts of social cognition is present in *yoga sutras.* Patanjali's description on *anumāna* (a tool for acquiring knowledge) is similar to what modern social psychology talk as ToM. The bias based approach in social psychology (unlike capacity based approach in psychology) fits well with the descriptions of Patanjali, that all that we perceive are colored by how do we perceive by our self.

# Chapter 3.0

# REVIEW OF SCIENTIFIC LITERATURE

# 3.0 REVIEW OF SCIENTIFIC LITERATURE

## 3.1 SCHIZOPHRENIA

Schizophrenia is a chronic psychotic disorder with cognitive, behavioural and emotional dysfunction. It's diagnosed as per DSM 5 (American Psychiatric Association, 2013a) with the following criteria,

1. Two (or more) of the following, each present for a significant portion of time during a 1-month period (or less if successfully treated). At least one of these must be (1), (2), or (3):

    1. Delusions.
    2. Hallucinations.
    3. Disorganized speech (e.g., frequent derailment or incoherence).
    4. Grossly disorganized or catatonic behavior.
    5. Negative symptoms (i.e., diminished emotional expression or avolition).

2. For a significant portion of the time since the onset of the disturbance, level of functioning in one or more major areas, such as work, interpersonal relations, or self-care, is markedly below the level achieved prior to the onset (or when the onset is in childhood or adolescence, there is failure to achieve expected level of interpersonal, academic, or occupational functioning).

3. Continuous signs of the disturbance persist for at least 6 months. This 6-month period must include at least 1 month of symptoms (or less if successfully treated) that meet Criterion A (i.e., active-phase symptoms) and may include periods of prodromal or residual symptoms. During these prodromal or residual periods, the signs of the disturbance may be manifested by only negative symptoms or by two or more symptoms listed in Criterion A present in an attenuated form (e.g., odd beliefs, unusual perceptual experiences).

4. Schizoaffective disorder and depressive or bipolar disorder with psychotic features have been ruled out because either 1) no major depressive or manic episodes have occurred concurrently with the active-phase symptoms, or 2) if mood episodes have occurred during active-phase symptoms, they have been present for a minority of the total duration of the active and residual periods of the illness.

5. The disturbance is not attributable to the physiological effects of a substance (e.g., a drug of abuse, a medication) or another medical condition.

6. If there is a history of autism spectrum disorder or a communication disorder of childhood onset, the additional diagnosis of schizophrenia is made only if prominent delusions or hallucinations, in addition to the other required symptoms of schizophrenia, are also present for at least 1 month (or less if successfully treated).

## 3.2 COGNITION

The term 'cognition' refers to many different processes by which individuals understand and make sense of the world. Social cognition concerns the various psychological processes that enable individuals to take advantage of being part of a social group(Frith & Frith, 2008). Brothers defined social cognition as the "mental operations underlying social interactions, which include the human ability and capacity to perceive the intentions and dispositions of others" (Brothers, 1990).

Broadly cognition can be classified as neurocognition (which includes attention, executive function, learning & memory, language & perceptual motor function) and social cognition.

## 3.3 SOCIAL COGNITION & ITS DOMAINS

Social cognition has not been studied widely among patient population until recently when a NIMH workshop consensus statement came up with various domains of social cognition and its application in research.

The NIMH workshop defined social cognition as "the mental operations that underlie social interactions, including perceiving, interpreting, and generating responses to the intentions, dispositions, and behaviours of others. As per the NIMH workshop consensus statement (Green et al., 2008), significant domains under which different items are grouped for clinical and research utility for social cognition that are applied frequently are a) Theory of mind, b) emotion processing, c) attributional styles and d) social perception & social knowledge.

These social cognition domains, their method of assessment and the neural correlates are described briefly in the following section including Mirror Neuron Activity (MNA), a phenomenon closely related to social cognition.

***Theory of Mind (ToM)***

Theory of Mind is the ability to infer the intentions and beliefs of others (Premack & Woodruff, 1978). ToM is also referred by various names as mentalizing, mental state attribution and social intelligence. This ToM capacity usually develops around the age of 4-5 years normally. ToM is assessed very commonly with simple short written stories of people interacting with each other with the subject asked to infer the intention or mental state of the people involved in the conversation. It can also be tested with short videos of geometrical shapes interacting with each other.

*Different levels of ToM*

ToM can be of varying complexity as follows,

1$^{st}$ order: The capacity to infer "*A* believes that *x*"

2$^{nd}$ order: The capacity to infer "*A* believes that *B* believes that *x*"

Stories with social blunders (Faux Pas and irony) are also considered as higher order ToM.

*ToM assessment*

Most of the literature available on ToM are in children comparing the normal and abnormal development of ToM. These ToM measures used in children with autism has been extended to patients with schizophrenia as well, due to similarity of social dysfunction in autism and schizophrenia. Though most of the studies assessing ToM in adult patients has used false belief task developed for children, there are some measures developed for use in adults specifically, like The Awareness of Social Inference Test (TASIT)(McDonald, Flanagan, Rollins, & Kinch, 2003), reading the mind in the eyes test (Eyes test)(Baron-Cohen, Wheelwright, Hill, Raste, & Plumb, 2001), etc.

*Brain regions involved in ToM*

Several brain regions involving medial prefrontal cortex (mPFC)(Amodio & Frith, 2006), bilateral temporoparietal junction (TPJ)(Mitchell, Heatherton, & Macrae, 2002) and precuneus were found to be activated during ToM task in healthy adults. Superior Temporal Sulcus (STS) and inferior frontal gyrus (IFG) are also activated in ToM task involving geometrical shape and inferring emotions from eyes respectively(Heider & Simmel, 1944).

***Emotional Processing (EP)***

Emotional processing is about perceiving and using emotions adaptively(Green & Horan, 2010). Emotions could be perceived through face, voice and bodily gestures. According to an influential model proposed by Salovey and colleagues emotional processing has four components which includes identifying emotions, facilitating emotions, understanding emotions and managing emotions(Mayer & Salovey, 1995). Face perception (affective and non-affective) and voice perception are also used to study emotion processing.

*Emotional Processing assessment*

Face perception is very commonly used tool for emotional perception. It's also an important aspect of social cue perception. Non-affective face perception involves processing of non-emotional information from the face like the age, sex or identity of a person. Affective face perception involves processing the emotions expressed in face of others.

Another tool which is a part of MATRICS cognitive battery is Mayer Salovey Caruso Emotional Intelligence Test or MSCEIT(Mayer, Salovey, Caruso, & Sitarenios, 2003). With this tool emotional processing is assessed in the following 4 abilities or branches: perceiving emotions, using emotions to facilitate thinking, understanding emotions, and managing emotions.

*Brain regions involved in emotional processing*

Affective face perception is associated with increased activation in limbic regions (amygdala, Parahippocampal gyrus and posterior cingulate cortex), inferior frontal gyrus (IFG), medial prefrontal gyrus and putamen (Fusar-Poli et al., 2009)(Vuilleumier & Pourtois, 2007)

Non- affective face perception is associated with increased activation in the bilateral fusiform face area (FFA; also known as lateral fusiform gyrus), visual extrastriate cortex, lateral occipital gyri, anterior temporal pole and posterior superior temporal gyrus (pSTG)(Fairhall & Ishai, 2007)(Gauthier et al., 2000)

Voice perception could be related to identity of the speaker, content/comprehension of the speech and affect of the content(Belin, Bestelmeyer, Latinus, & Watson, 2011). Anterior temporal-lobe regions of the right hemisphere, particularly right anterior STS regions, are associated in processing information related to speaker identity. Affective nonverbal vocalizations such as laughs, cries, groans are associated with activation of amygdala and anterior insula. Right temporal lobe and right inferior prefrontal cortex activation is associated with perceiving emotions from the prosody of speech. Comprehension of the speech is found to activate anterior regions of the left STS/superior temporal plane(Belin, Fecteau, & Bédard, 2004)

***Attribution Style (AS)***

Attribution bias or style refers to the manner in which individuals interpret, explain, or make sense of the positive and negative social events encountered in life and is thought to have a significant impact on behaviours(Green et al., 2008). Attributional bias may be external personal attributions (i.e. causes attributed to other people), external situational attributions (i.e. causes attributed to situational factors), and internal attributions (i.e. causes due to oneself). There are numerous factors which influences the attribution style including the actor's intention, perceiver's motivation and cultural differences.

Based on whether the attribution style favours the perceiver's motive or intention, attribution could be a categorized as self-serving bias/personalizing bias and externalizing bias(Bentall, Corcoran, Howard, Blackwood, &

Kinderman, 2001)(Combs, Penn, Wicher, & Waldheter, 2007). Attributing positive events to the self or negative events to others is self-serving bias and the vice versa is externalizing bias

Various models have been proposed for explaining the process of attribution. The most influential being the three-stage model proposed by Gilbert & colleagues(Gilbert, Krull, & Pelham, 1988). This three-stage model includes,

a) categorization/identification stage

b) characterization stage

c) correction stage

Categorization stage is identifying the cues of target, situation and cues experienced from the target person in past. Characterization involves a correspondent dispositional inference which is automatic/reflexive and correction stage involves a reflective stage where the dispositional inference is adjusted for the situational forces.

*Attribution style assessment*

Assessment of attribution style dates back to the beginning of social cognition in the in 1940s with the classical film created by Heider and Simmel (1944)(Heider & Simmel, 1944) of geometrical shapes moving against a white background.

The most commonly used tool is Internal Personal Situational Attribution Style Questionnaire-IPSAQ (an extension of Attribution Style Questionnaire-ASQ)(Kinderman & Bentall, 1996). IPSAQ gives a set of imaginary situations for which the subject has to attribute the causes-external (personal/ situational) or internal

*Brain regions involved in attribution*

As attribution involves both automatic and reflexive processing, it is speculated that corresponding brain regions might be activated(Gilbert, 1989). For example, when dispositional inference is adjusted for the situational factors, prefrontal cortex is found to be associated with this correction stage of attribution process. This is further supported by studies which has demonstrated the disruption in correction dispositional inference stage by the cognitive demand of daily lives like making a positive impression(Gilbert & Malone, 1995). During automatic processing stage of attribution lateral temporal cortex and superior temporal sulcus are involved.

***Social perception(SP) and social knowledge***

Social perception is the ability to judge social roles and rules in a social context(Corrigan & Green, 1993a). Social perception overlaps with two other areas - emotion perception and social knowledge.

Though similar to emotion perception, it differs in the type of judgement. In social perception, social cues are inferred to situational events that generated the cue unlike emotion perception where emotional qualities are inferred from facial expression or voice tone.

Social knowledge is about the roles and rules that characterize a specific social situation(Corrigan, Wallace, & Green, 1992). Example- role of a doctor in clinic, role of a waiter in a restaurant. Social knowledge overlaps with social perception as some amount of social knowledge is required for appropriate social perception.

*Social perception & social knowledge assessment*

Social perception is assessed with short video clips of 2-3 people interacting with each other. Subjects is supposed to answer set of questions from the video clips inferring about the rules, affect and the roles guiding the person's behaviour. Social Cue Recognition test (SCRT)(Corrigan & Green, 1993a) is the tool commonly used for social perception assessment.

Social knowledge is a paper and pencil measure in which the participants are asked to identify some features from a list of descriptors that define a familiar situation. It's assessed using the Situational Features Recognition Test (SFRT)(Corrigan & Green, 1993b)

*Brain regions associated with social perception and social knowledge*

Ventromedial prefrontal cortex has been implicated in social knowledge and behaviour especially in brain injury studies in primates and human beings. In humans lesions of ventromedial prefrontal cortex are associated with difficulty in incorporating emotional information in to the social context and make social reasoning and judgement. Adolph has reported that patients with prefrontal lesions were more accurate in reasoning from a non-social scenario than a social scenario compared to the comparison subjects(Adolphs, 1999).

***Mirror Neuron Activity (MNA)***

Mirror neuron system is a specialized network of neurons which are activated when one performs an action as well as when he / she observes such action and it is an underlying process of all social interactions(Di Pellegrino, Fadiga, Fogassi, Gallese, & Rizzolatti, 1992).

Recently it has been speculated as a mediator for automatic cognitive processing in the Dual Processing(DP) theory of social cognition.

*MNA Assessment*

Mirror neuron activity has been demonstrated by direct method, single-cell electrode recordings (Mukamel, Ekstrom, Kaplan, Iacoboni, & Fried, 2010) and indirect methods such as, functional magnetic resonance imaging or functional MRI (fMRI) (Rizzolatti & Craighero, 2004), electroencephalogram (EEG) (Pineda & Hecht, 2009) (Oberman, Ramachandran, & Pineda, 2008) magnetoencephalography(MEG) (Kato et al., 2011) and transcranial magnetic stimulation (TMS) (Mehta, Basavaraju, Thirthalli, & Gangadhar, 2012). Functional Near Infra Red Spectroscopy fNIRS) is an emerging technique of brain imaging to study cortical responses measured by hemodynamic variations. fNIRS has also been used in assessing MNA in a recent study with Pervasive Developmental Disorders(PDD)(Kajiume, Aoyama-Setoyama, Saito-Hori, Ishikawa, & Kobayashi, 2013). Different indirect methods of MNA assessment are as follows,

**Table-3.1 MNA assessment-indirect methods**

| S.No | Method | Putative measure of MNA |
|---|---|---|
| 1 | fMRI | Blood oxygenation level–dependent changes |

| | | |
|---|---|---|
| 2 | TMS | Motor evoked potential (MEP) Enhancement |
| 3 | EEG | mu Rhythm suppression |
| 4 | PET | Blood flow changes & Glucose metabolism |
| 5 | MEG | Alpha band suppression and gamma band amplifications |
| 6 | fNIRS | Blood oxygenation level–dependent changes |

*Brain regions associated with MNA*

Specific sets of temporal, parietal and frontal areas contribute to different aspects of MNA in human beings.

The overall mirror neuron circuitry of humans is composed of core circuit of premotor cortex and parietal (posterior parietal lobule) cortex containing the mirror neurons (Rizzolatti & Craighero, 2004), and visual cortex of the temporal lobe (posterior temporal sulcus) intimately linked to these two areas. The visual cortex of the temporal lobe provides visual input to the core mirror areas and also receives information about motor intentions (Iacoboni et al., 2005).

## 3.4 COGNITIVE DEFICIT IN SCHIZOPHRENIA

People with schizophrenia generally perform 1.5 to 2 standard deviations below the healthy normal people in cognitive (neurocognition) function tests (Saykin & Gur, 1991). Patients with schizophrenia show impairment in most of the domains of neuro-cognition and social cognition. Social cognition deficits are present in schizophrenia patients even when in remission (Mehta, Bhagyavathi, Thirthalli, Kumar, & Gangadhar, 2014).

## 3.5 COGNITIVE DEFICIT AND FUNCTIONAL OUTCOME IN SCHIZOPHRENIA

Cognitive deficits both neurocognition and social cognition has been very well documented in schizophrenia (Fett, Viechtbauer, Dominguez, et al., 2011). Indeed, social cognitive deficits play a key role in determining the functional outcome including social and vocational capacities in schizophrenia (Fig-3.1). Social cognitive abilities make one interact effectively in social environment and lack of social cognition might lead to poor or maladaptive understanding and experience of the social situations leading to social withdrawal(D. L. Penn, Sanna, & Roberts, 2008). Studying social cognitive deficit would also enable us to understand the clinical symptoms like paranoia and negative symptoms much better.

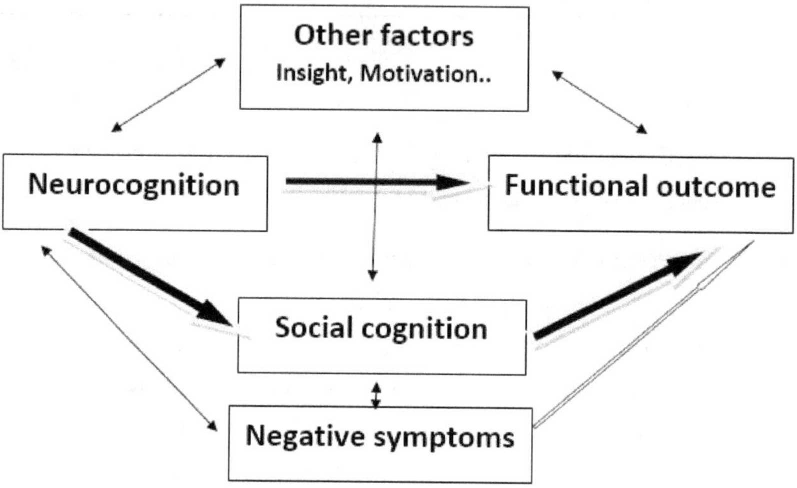


**Figure-3.1 Social cognition & functional outcome**

## 3.6 SOCIAL COGNITIVE DEFICIT IN SCHIZOPHRENIA

Social cognition is an emerging topic in the field of mental health. Though research on attribution (mostly on healthy population) formed the core for social cognition development in the beginning, its recent application in diseased population has brought out different domains which are evolving progressively over time with emerging empirical evidences. For example, the same four domains of social cognition-ToM, EP, AS and SP were organized conceptually in a little different way by Green et al (Green, Horan, & Lee, 2015) in a recent review, with some more additions like, MNA, empathy, etc under the same umbrella theme of social cognition.

The following section gives details of social cognition deficit based on the conceptual framework of Green et al (2015).

But, before going to details of social cognition deficit in schizophrenia, it would be useful to understand the theoretical model of social cognition.

***Model for understanding social cognition***

One of the most influential model in social cognition is the Dual Processing (DP) theory (Evans, 2008). The dual processing framework views social cognitive judgements as results of interaction between the automatic and controlled cognitive processing (Chaiken & Trope, 1999).

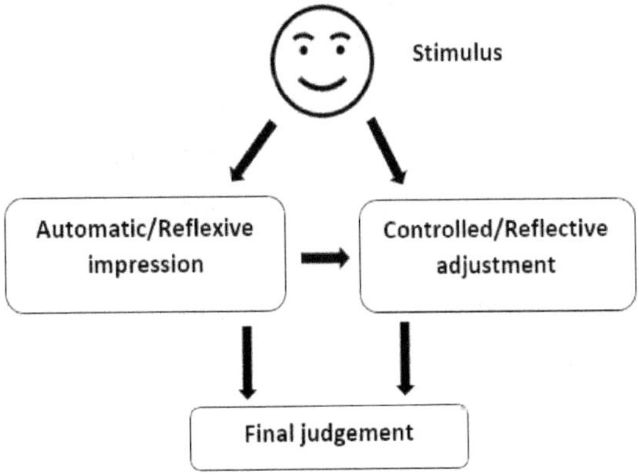


**Fig- 3.2 Dual Processing (DP) theory of social cognition**

Automatic processing is the primary mechanism for generating initial social cognitive representation, which may later be manipulated as per the need of the self & situation. It is fast and efficient and largely happens outside of one's conscious awareness. Automatic generation of social cognitive representations draws on early perception-based representations of others' facial features and bodily motion, mediated in part by fusiform gyrus and superior temporal sulcus, respectively. It also draws on well-rehearsed interpersonal scripts or stereotypes, and emotional experiences and representations of the subject's own bodily and physiological states, as mediated by subcortical structures such as the amygdala and insula (Lieberman, 2007). Actual neural mechanisms by which automatic process sub serves the heuristic manipulations and hence the automatic social cognitive representations are not understood. One speculation that gained empirical support in recent years is mirror neuron system (Carr, Iacoboni, Dubeau, Mazziotta, & Lenzi, 2003).

Controlled processing is the capacity to consciously manipulate the cognitive representations, allowing the subject to strategically evaluate, modify or suppress the automatic impressions which are maladaptive or inconsistent with the subject's goals.

The basic DP model of social cognition is illustrated in figure 3.2. Automatic processing responds immediately to a social stimulus, quickly and unconsciously generating an actionable impression on the basis of whatever combination of perceptions, emotion, cognitive schemas, and physiological inputs happen to be most salient at the time. After roughly 500 ms post stimulus onset, controlled processing may or may not be engaged to modify or suppress this initial impression, depending on multiple factors. Controlled processing is less likely to be engaged if the automatic impression is highly salient; if the subject is experiencing cognitive load, emotional arousal, or distraction; is cognitively impaired; is unaware that the initial impression may be maladaptive; or is not motivated to question the initial impression. Failure to actively engage controlled cognition results in passive endorsement of the automatic impression, and subsequent controlled processing will be biased toward its continued endorsement.

### *Applying the Dual-Process Framework to Social Cognition in Schizophrenia*

The social cognitive deficits in schizophrenia can be conceptualized in the light of dual processing framework as follows,

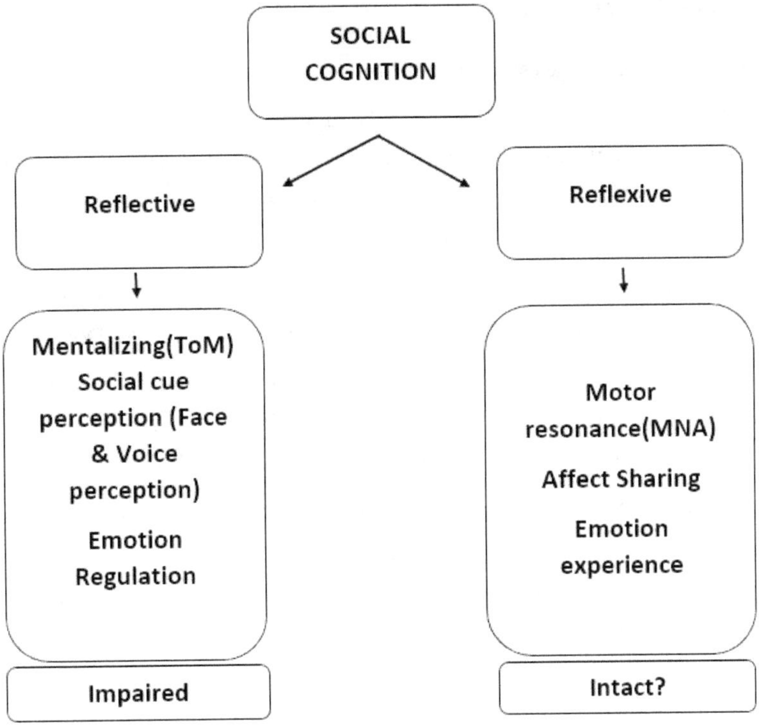


**Fig-3.3 Social cognitive deficits in schizophrenia in the light of DP framework**

Social cognitive abnormality in schizophrenia results from two factors:

(1) diminished controlled processing capacity and

(2) excessively salient and aberrant automatic social cognitive impressions.

There is broad support in the literature for the first factor, as schizophrenia is linked to diminished prefrontal functioning (Ragland, Yoon, Minzenberg, & Carter, 2007). There is also support for the second factor in the literature on dopamine-mediated aberrant salience experience (Kapur, Mizrahi, & Li, 2005), including evidence that dysregulated neural signalling causes feelings of social threat, alien control, and other forms of aberrant intentionality. This two-factor model predicts the generation of highly salient but maladaptively biased automatic social cognitive impressions (e.g., the impression of being the object of hostility) in combination with a handicapped ability to evaluate, suppress, or modify these dysfunctional impressions.

### *Mentalizing (ToM) Deficit*

Neuroimaging studies showed that patients with SCZ had decreased activity in some core regions of the mentalizing system. During a task that required subjects to use the perspectives of others to correctly identify objects, patients showed reduced activation of the ventromedial PFC (vmPFC) and orbitofrontal cortex (Eack, Wojtalik, Newhill, Keshavan, & Phillips, 2013).Patients also showed decreased activation of the mPFC and TPJ while making inferences about the beliefs of others (Lee, Quintana, Nori, & Green, 2011) (Dodell-Feder, Tully, Lincoln, & Hooker, 2014). Controls showed less activation in the mentalizing system when inferring the intentions of a person in isolation compared with inferring the intentions of a person who is participating in a social interaction, and patients failed to show this modulation (Walter et al., 2009). Another study found that, compared with controls, people with schizophrenia exhibited increased activity in the superior temporal gyrus (STG), dorsomedial PFC (dmPFC) and precuneus when inferring the intentions of others (Brüne et al., 2008). In both of these studies, the individuals with schizophrenia showed intact performance, suggesting that they required greater levels of neural activity to achieve the same levels of performance on mentalizing tasks as controls.

To summarize, the patterns of aberrant activation on mentalizing tasks are not consistent across studies. Most studies report hypoactivation of the core mentalizing system and impaired mentalizing ability in behavioural tasks. A few studies found hyperactivation of brain regions associated with mentalizing. Individuals with schizophrenia may need greater activation in these regions to achieve the same level of mentalizing proficiency, suggesting neural inefficiency – potential to result in delayed activation of this network.

### *Non-affective face perception*

Patients with schizophrenia have less difficulty with coarse judgments of facial features but have more difficulty with finer-grained judgments (Darke, Peterman, Park, Sundram, & Carter, 2013) (Bortolon, Capdevielle, & Raffard, 2015). Individuals with and without schizophrenia have similar levels of neural activation in the FFA during non-affective face perception (Walther et al.,

2009). Patterns of neural activation across FFA voxels during a non-affective face-perception task were less cohesive in patients with schizophrenia (Yoon, D'Esposito, & Carter, 2006).

### *Affective face perception*

Individuals with schizophrenia show less activation in the right inferior occipital gyrus, right fusiform gyrus, left amygdala and hippocampal regions, anterior cingulate cortex (ACC), medial prefrontal cortex (mPFC) and thalamus. However, they show greater activation in the insula, cuneus, parietal lobule and STG during affective face perception (Li, Chan, McAlonan, & Gong, 2009) (Taylor et al., 2012) (Delvecchio, Sugranyes, & Frangou, 2013). Blunted response in the amygdala seen in individuals with schizophrenia during contrasts of emotional versus neutral conditions might be due to increased activation in response to neutral stimuli (Anticevic et al., 2010). Studies using ERP to assess neural activation during face perception have focused on two components:

1) N170 at occipitotemporal sites, which is associated with structural information of
faces (Bentin, Allison, Puce, Perez, & McCarthy, 1996)
2) N250 at frontocentral sites, which is associated with facial emotional information (Marinkovic & Halgren, 1998).

A meta-analysis of various schizophrenia studies revealed robust deficits in N170 and N250 components during affective face perception (McCleery et al., 2015).

To summarize, studies of non-affective face processing in schizophrenia have yielded conflicting results, whereas studies of affective face processing in schizophrenia are more consistent. Patients with schizophrenia demonstrate hypoactivation in brain regions associated with affective face perception and hyperactivation in regions not typically associated with face perception. Patients may recruit other areas to compensate for dysfunction in the key face-processing regions.

### *Voice perception*

These are acoustic properties of speech that provide critical information beyond the meaning of words or grammatical structure, such as emotional state, emphasis, contrasts and focuses. Findings of non-affective prosody in schizophrenia are mixed, in that patients correctly perceive certain features of non-affective prosody and have difficulties with perceiving pitch and rhythm. Studies on affective prosody perception have shown consistent behavioural impairment, and the few neuroimaging studies carried out to date suggest hypoactivation in key regions, for example, the STG and IFG.

***Emotion regulation***

The emotion regulation system influences expression of emotions within appropriate social contexts and includes brain regions that overlap with the amygdala and the ventral and dorsal lateral prefrontal cortices. Dysfunctional neural activity in these brain regions has regularly been demonstrated in schizophrenia.

In two fMRI studies schizophrenia patients showed ventro-lateral prefrontal cortex hypoactivation while emotional responses were decreased and vlPFC hyperactivation while emotional responses were increased. Neural activity in the amygdala was inversely coupled with prefrontal activation activation in controls, but not in those with schizophrenia (Morris, Sparks, Mitchell, Weickert, & Green, 2012) (van der Meer et al., 2014)

To summarize, converging evidence suggests that the use of cognitive reappraisal strategies is disrupted in schizophrenia, a conclusion that is consistent with the neural impairments in cognitive control processes in this disorder (Nuechterlein, Luck, Lustig, & Sarter, 2009) (Carter, Bowling, Reeck, & Huettel, 2012) . The interface between cognitive control and emotional processes is an active area of translational research in schizophrenia.

***Motor resonance/MNA***

Evidence available for MNA in schizophrenia is mixed, which is listed as follows,

*fMRI studies:*

Two fMRI studies of motor resonance in schizophrenia have provided conflicting results. Patients with schizophrenia showed decreased activation in the right inferior parietal lobule (IPL) and posterior superior temporal sulcus (STS) during action observation, but increased activation in these regions during imitation of finger movements (Thakkar, Peterman, & Park, 2014). Patients and controls showed similar activation in the expected brain regions across conditions, including inferior frontal, premotor and inferior parietal cortices, suggesting intact motor resonance in schizophrenia (Horan, Pineda, Wynn, Iacoboni, & Green, 2014).

*TMS studies:*

Two TMS studies yielded mixed findings, showing evidence of either diminished or intact mirror neuron system activation (Enticott et al., 2008) (Mehta, Thirthalli, Basavaraju, Gangadhar, & Pascual-Leone, 2013).

*EEG studies:*

'Mu' wave suppression: - Suppression of mu during observation and execution of actions has been found and is thought to be a physiological index of mirror neuron system activity. Three studies found no differences in mu suppression between individuals with schizophrenia and healthy subjects (McCormick et al., 2012) (Singh, Pineda, & Cadenhead, 2011) (Horan et al., 2014). But one study found diminished mu suppression in patients compared with healthy controls (Mitra, Nizamie, Goyal, & Tikka, 2014).

*MEG studies:*

Two small MEG studies reported diminished mirror neuron system activity in individuals with schizophrenia compared with healthy controls and with healthy co-twins (SchÜrmann et al., 2007) (Kato et al., 2011).

To summarize, the findings from motor resonance studies of schizophrenia are mixed. This area of research is still relatively new and the scientific approaches used are highly diverse, which may account for some of the discrepancies in the findings.

***Affect sharing***

Neural activation in certain limbic regions, particularly the amygdala, insula and cingulate gyrus occurs when an individual executes facial expressions of emotion and when an individual observes another person making such expressions. Studies of affect sharing have also focused on the perception of others when they display physical pain. Studies in healthy people demonstrate that the anterior insula and dorsal ACC, which are involved in the affective and motivational processing of schizophrenia, are also activated by the observation of others' pain (Lamm, Decety, & Singer, 2011).In self-report studies, patients score similarly to healthy controls for personal traits associated with affect sharing, and some showed tendency to be overly sensitive and reactive to the feelings of others compared with healthy controls (Michaels et al., 2014). Patients and controls showed a similar pattern of mu suppression in response to stimuli depicting various social interactions (Horan et al., 2014).In another study, individuals with recent-onset schizophrenia showed normal mu suppression for stimuli depicting social interaction stimuli, although they displayed diminished mu suppression while viewing stimuli depicting human biological motion. (Singh et al., 2011). Early event related potential (ERP)-processing components (N110, P180 and N240) during an affect-sharing task both patients and healthy controls showed similar levels of sensitivity to pain relevant stimuli (Corbera, Ikezawa, Bell, & Wexler, 2014). In a fMRI study, although imitation and execution of emotional expressions were impaired in patients, both groups showed similar levels of activation in regions associated with affect sharing, including inferior prefrontal, premotor, and inferior and superior parietal cortices (Horan et al., 2014)

To summarize, several studies using various methods report normal, or even enhanced, affect sharing in schizophrenia. Thus, affect sharing may reflect a relatively preserved aspect of social cognition in schizophrenia.

***Emotion experience***

Emotion experience activates the amygdala, anterior hippocampus, ACC and anterior insula. Emotion experience in schizophrenia is largely intact during exposure to both pleasant and unpleasant stimuli (Horan, Foti, Hajcak, Wynn,

& Green, 2012) (Pinheiro et al., 2013).The capacity to effectively regulate negative emotions would therefore be critical for normal adaptive functioning in schizophrenia.

***Attribution style in schizophrenia***

Individuals with persecutory delusions often attribute negative outcomes to others, rather than situations. This is known as a personalizing bias (Bentall et al., 2001). Similarly, schizophrenia patients also found to have hostile attributional biases or the tendency to attribute hostile intentions to others' actions (Combs, Penn, et al., 2007).

## 3.7 SUMMARY OF SOCIAL COGNITIVE DEFICIT IN SCHIZOPHRENIA

From the behavioural and neuroscientific studies discussed above, we can conclude that there is strong evidence to suggest that people with schizophrenia have impairments in some, but not all, social processes. There is consistent evidence to suggest schizophrenia is associated with impairments in face and prosody perception, mentalizing and emotion regulation. By contrast, the findings regarding emotion experience in schizophrenia suggest that this process is largely intact. In addition, some evidence suggests that motor resonance and affect sharing are intact in schizophrenia. However, it is important to note that there are relatively few studies on experience sharing to date and that some of the findings of these studies are inconsistent; hence, it is difficult to make firm conclusions. Nonetheless, the available data suggest that any impairment in experience sharing may be subtle.

Another interesting observation is, all the social cognitive process which are reflective are impaired but not the reflexive social cognitive process.

## 3.8 BRAIN REGIONS ASSOCIATED WITH SOCIAL COGNITION DEFICIT IN SCHIZOPHRENIA

Social cognition can be divided into several distinct processes, which involve many different brain regions, some of which show overlap between processes. Perceiving social cues incorporates face perception, which is associated with activation of the amygdala and fusiform face area (FFA), and voice perception, which activates the superior temporal gyrus (STG) and inferior frontal gyrus (IFG). Experience sharing includes the processes of motor resonance, which activates the inferior

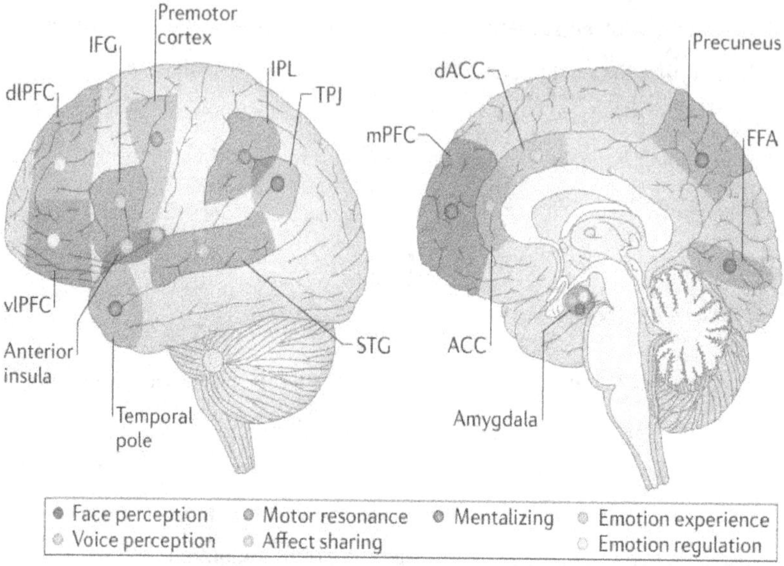


**Fig-3.4 Brain regions in social process (from Green et al, 2015)**

parietal lobule (IPL) and premotor cortex, and affect sharing, which activates the dorsal anterior cingulate cortex (dACC) and anterior insula. Mentalizing activates various regions, including the temporoparietal junction (TPJ), temporal pole, precuneus and medial prefrontal cortex (mPFC). Emotion experience activates the amygdala, anterior hippocampus (not shown), ACC and anterior insula, and emotion regulation activates brain regions including the dorsolateral PFC (dlPFC), ventrolateral PFC (vlPFC) and amygdala. These brain regions and associated social processes are not entirely separate; for example, the anterior insula is involved in both affect sharing and emotion experience, and the amygdala is involved in face perception, emotion experience and emotion regulation. Note that these regions are a representative, but not comprehensive, listing of relevant brain regions for each social cognitive process.

## 3.9 MNA AND SOCIAL COGNITIVE DEFICIT-THE RELATIONSHIP

In recent years, theories have come up trying to place MNA as one of the key contributor for social cognition. For example, ToM is explained based on one of the theories called simulation theory. Simulation theory is based on the fact that we are able to understand others intuitively, as we all have similar kind of representations within ourselves. With this theory, MNA goes hand in hand with ToM. There is recent speculation that MNA might underlie the automatic processing of social cognitive representation, as per the DP theory of social cognition (Carr et al., 2003).

Similarly, the neural correlates of empathy include inferior frontal gyrus (IFG), right superior temporal sulcus (STS), right inferior parietal lobe (IPL), anterior cingulate cortex (ACC), ventromedial prefrontal cortex (VMPFC), somatosensory cortex, amygdala, precuneus, insula and the posterior cingulate. Thus, empathy involves a significant interaction of the core MNS and its limbic extension (Iacoboni, 2005).

In summary, considering social cognition in the context of social learning through imitation, there is emerging evidence to speculate MNA as a key contributor of social cognition.

## 3.10 TREATMENT FOR COGNITIVE DYSFUNCTION

Most of the biological treatments work better for the positive symptoms of schizophrenia, but not for the negative symptoms or the cognitive dysfunction (Szöke, Trandafir, Dupont, Méary, Schürhoff, Schu, et al., 2008) (Moncrieff, 2011).Social cognition deficits persist despite antipsychotic treatment.

***Interventions for social cognitive deficit***

Social cognition training is not a new comer in the area of psychosocial rehabilitation. Its origin can be traced back to social skills training and neurocognitive remediation.

Although social skills training and neurocognitive remediation has the same goal of improving social and community functioning, the targets are different in these programs. Social skills training program were developed based on social learning theory and operant conditioning techniques and focuses mainly on motor behaviours like eye contact, speech content, duration and loudness, whereas neurocognitive remediation focuses on attention, memory and problem solving. (as literature shows significant link between neurocognition and various functioning)

Concept of social cognition training is a combination of both social skills and basic cognition training. Nonetheless, there are various manual based training programs for improving the community and social functioning targeting only social domains (few domains or comprehensive) with or without neurocognitive training.

Accordingly, social cognitive training programs can be broadly classified as

1) Targeted treatments

2) Comprehensive treatments

3) Broad based treatment approaches

**Table-3.2 Social cognitive training programs**

| S. No | Treatments | Approach | Focus |
|---|---|---|---|
| 1 | Training in Affect Recognition (TAR) | Targeted | Affect perception |
| 2 | Social Cognition Enhancement Training (SCET) | Targeted | Social perception |
| 3 | Emotion & ToM Imitation Training(ETIT) | Targeted | ToM & Emotion processing |
| 4 | Social Cognition Interaction Training(SCIT) | Comprehensive | Full range of Social cognition |

| | | | |
|---|---|---|---|
| 5 | Social Cognition Skills Training(SCST) | Comprehensive | Similar to SCIT with add-on TAR |
| 6 | Meta Cognitive Therapy (MCT) | Comprehensive | ToM, Attribution, Memory & Cognitive biases |
| 7 | Integrated Psychological Therapy (IPT) | Broad based | Basic cognitive (CBT based) & social cognitive remediation with psychosocial rehabilitation |
| 8 | Cognitive Enhancement Therapy(CET) | Broad based | Social cognition with neurocognition |
| 9 | Integrated Neurological Therapy (INT) | Broad based | Social cognition & Neurocognition with MATRICS defined domains |

Brief descriptions of available treatments for social cognitive deficit:

*Training in Affect Recognition (TAR)*

TAR is a 6-week, 12-session, manualized treatment consisting of three segments: identification of prototypical components of basic emotions, integration of facial elements to form quick decisions about affect, and application of learned information to the processing of non-prototypical, ambiguous facial expressions. The training relies on both compensatory and restorative techniques, includes both computerized stimuli and "desk work," and relies heavily on strategies like verbalization and self-instruction.

In an efficacy trial of TAR, Wolwer and colleagues (Wölwer et al., 2005) randomly assigned 77 post-acute schizophrenia inpatients and outpatients to TAR, cognitive remediation therapy (CRT), or treatment as usual (TAU). CRT consisted of 12 sessions of computerized training in attention, memory, and executive function, as well as dyad training in cognitive strategies. An intent-to-treat analyses, the authors reported significant group differences in affect recognition and basic neurocognitive performance. Individuals in the TAR group improved significantly more than the other two groups on pre–post measures of affect recognition, whereas individuals in CRT improved significantly more than TAU on measures of memory and learning.

*Social Cognition Enhancement Training (SCET)*

Social Cognition Enhancement Training (SCET) (Choi & Kwon, 2006), which focuses on improving social context appraisal and perspective-taking abilities through practice with arranging cartoons of social situations, has been shown to improve social perception, although the training did not generalize to affect recognition.

Van der Gaag and colleagues (van der Gaag, Kern, van den Bosch, & Liberman, 2002) have also evaluated the efficacy of a social perception combined with emotion recognition training. Evaluated in a sample of 42 inpatients with schizophrenia randomized to either the treatment or time-matched leisure activities, the training led to improvements in social perception, with a 23% reduction in errors on emotion matching and a 49% reduction in errors on emotion labelling. There was also some evidence of improvements in executive function; however, these were only observed in within- group paired t-tests.

*Emotion & ToM Imitation Training (ETIT)*

Roncone and colleagues (Roncone et al., 2004) randomly assigned 20 inpatients with residual schizophrenia to Instrumental Enrichment Program (IEP) or a usual treatment control condition. IEP, which the authors compare to Hogarty and colleagues' Cognitive Enhancement Therapy, focuses on exposing participants to new situations and decreasing ToM impairments by "teaching and learning how to change cognitive structure by transforming a passive dependent cognitive style to an autonomous one".

IEP was conducted in a single 6-month weekly group, which included ten patients and five therapists. Compared to the control condition, IEP was associated with decreases in negative symptoms, improvements in ToM (both first- and second-order false beliefs), executive functions, strategic thinking, and affect recognition for two types of emotions—sadness and fear.

In another study of the malleability of ToM impairments, Mazza and colleagues (Mazza et al., 2010) compared changes in ToM performance following 12 sessions of Emotion and ToM Imitation Training (ETIT) or Problem-Solving Skill Training (PST) administered to 33 outpatients with schizophrenia. ETIT is a group-based treatment consisting of four training phases: observing others' eye direction, imitating facial emotions, inferring others' mental states, and making attributions of intentions based on observations of others' actions. Compared to the active control condition, individuals randomized to ETIT evidenced improvements in several ToM measures, affect recognition, empathy, clinician-rated social functioning, and positive symptoms. Improvements in memory were observed only in the group receiving PST.

*Social Cognition Interaction Training (SCIT)*

Social Cognition and Interaction Training (SCIT) is a comprehensive, standalone manual-based group intervention that targets the three-core social cognitive deficits in schizophrenia: emotion perception, theory of mind (ToM), and attributional style (Roberts, Penn, Labate, Margolis, & Sterne, 2010).

SCIT is comprised of three distinct phases, lasts 20–24 weeks, and is built around a weekly 1-hour group therapy session. SCIT involves the use of didactic instruction, videotape and computerized learning tools, and role-play methods to improve social cognition. SCIT involves weekly homework assignments and uses optional phone-in contacts and practice partners to consolidate gains made in the sessions.

SCIT has shown improvements in both inpatients and outpatients with schizophrenia (Combs, Adams, et al., 2007) (D. Penn et al., 2005) (Roberts & Penn, 2009) and these gains persist at 6-month follow-up (Combs et al., 2009). SCIT has the potential to become an evidence based treatment for schizophrenia (D. L. Penn, Roberts, Combs, & Sterne, 2007).

*Social Cognition Skills Training (SCST)*

Social Cognitive Skill Training (SCST) was developed by Green, Horan, and colleagues at the University of California at Los Angeles (UCLA) and combines and expands on elements from other social cognitive treatments including SCIT and TAR.

In the first evaluation of the feasibility and tolerability of SCST (Horan et al., 2009), 34 schizophrenia spectrum outpatients, social cognitive training was associated with significant improvements in affect recognition, with large between-group and medium to large within-group effect sizes; these improvements were independent of any change in neurocognitive function or clinical symptoms. There were also trend-level improvements on measures of attributional bias and ToM.

In a subsequent evaluation of the now-expanded SCST treatment (Horan et al., 2011), 85 individuals with psychotic disorders were randomized to receive one of four time-matched treatments: SCST, computerized neurocognitive remediation, a hybrid intervention that included both SCST and neurocognitive remediation components, and a standard illness management skills training group. There were no significant between-group differences on measures of social perception, attributional bias, or ToM, nor on neurocognition or psychiatric symptoms. There was a trend-level improvement for social skill ability in both the SCST and the neurocognitive remediation group. But differential effects favouring SCST were found for affect recognition, which generalized to emotion management. Because effects on emotion processing were specific to the SCST group, the authors conclude that this intervention has a specific effect on social cognition not observed for the other three treatment conditions, and they suggest that efforts at improving social cognition may be successful in stand-alone social cognitive treatments that do not require concomitant neurocognitive remediation.

*Meta Cognitive Therapy (MCT)*

Metacognitive training (MCT; from metacognition, "thinking about one's thinking") is a novel approach founded in the tradition of psychoeducation, cognitive remediation, social cognition training and CBT. MCT targets cognitive biases putatively involved in delusion formation, for which patients often lack adequate awareness. Another explicit aim of MCT is to foster improved social cognition and theory of mind.

Various studies have asserted the feasibility of the MCT (S Moritz, Veckenstedt, Randjbar, Vitzthum, & Woodward, 2011) (Steffen Moritz & Woodward, 2007) in German and other languages. Researchers, have also shown a positive impact on symptoms (Aghotor, Pfueller, Moritz, Weisbrod, & Roesch-Ely, 2010) (Kumar et al., 2010) (Ross, Freeman, Dunn, & Garety, 2009). Although there is increasing support for the efficacy of the MCT as a stand-alone program, it is probably best to use it with along with other therapies like CBT.

*Integrated Psychological Therapy (IPT)*

IPT was one of the very first comprehensive and manual-driven group therapy approaches for schizophrenia patients. IPT is a "bottom-up" and "top-down" approach, addressing both basic cognitive building blocks and higher order integrative processing. It consists of five subprograms, each with incremental steps. IPT starts with a subprogram addressing the neurocognitive domain, followed by a second subprogram to enhance social cognition. In a third stage, IPT focuses on interpersonal and social context using verbal communication tools, thereby bridging the gap between cognitive and social functioning. Finally, social competence is targeted with exercises to improve social skills (fourth subprogram) and to increase patients' mastery in coping with interpersonal and social problems (fifth subprogram) for more independent living.

A meta-analysis of the efficacy of IPT (Roder, Mueller, Mueser, & Brenner, 2006), however, indicates efficacy in all examined domains, including neurocognition, psychiatric symptoms, and psychosocial functioning, with within-group effect sizes in the medium range. This pattern of findings persists when only methodologically rigorous IPT studies with large samples are included, and it generalizes to a broad range of assessment types, settings, and treatment phases. There is also evidence that the effects of IPT are maintained or even enhanced during an average follow-up period of over 8 months.

*Cognitive Enhancement Therapy(CET)*

CET is a broad-based psychosocial treatment combining neurocognitive remediation and social cognitive group training. Although from the beginning CET has been conceptualized as a social cognitive treatment, it nevertheless includes a significant neurocognitive training component, with neurocognition seen as a necessary building block for successful social behaviour.

In the first published evaluation of CET (Hogarty et al., 2004) with 121 chronically ill patients with schizophrenia randomized to 2 years of CET or an illness self-management focused intervention called Enriched Supportive Therapy (EST), group differences favouring CET were observed on processing speed, neurocognition, and social adjustment, with trend-level improvements for social cognition and cognitive style were observed at the end of one year.

At the end of the 2-year treatment, observed group differences remained or were enhanced, with large effect size improvements for CET on all assessed composite scores, with the exception of psychiatric symptoms. Most importantly perhaps, at the end of treatment, the groups differed significantly on measures of social functioning and social adjustment, including vocational and interpersonal effectiveness, instrumental task performance, and adjustment to disability. In an effort to disentangle relevant patient variables associated with treatment efficacy, the authors report that when the sample was divided into more versus less chronic patients (those ill for more or less than 15 years), among more chronic patients, CET participants improved more than EST participants only on measures of reaction time, whereas for the less chronic patients, group differences were observed on several of the assessed domains, including social functioning, suggesting that CET may be particularly helpful to individuals earlier in the course of illness.

In a subsequent report of the durability of CET effects 1-year after the conclusion of treatment (Hogarty, Greenwald, & Eack, 2006), follow-up data were available for close to 90% of the originally randomized sample. Posttreatment CET improvements were maintained on processing speed, cognitive style, social cognition, and social adjustment, and there was evidence that early (first year) improvements in processing speed mediated improvements in social cognition and social adjustment in the CET group. Perhaps of most interest is that at the follow-up assessment, group differences were noted on several real-world outcomes, including participation in social, recreational, or therapeutic group activities, with 30% of the CET group (vs. only 9% of EST group) engaged in these types of activities.

A similar kind of study (Eack, Greenwald, Hogarty, & Keshavan, 2010) with early course illness from the same researchers have shown results favouring the CET with maintenance of effect at one year follow up.

CET has also been reported to be associated with changes in brain morphology (Eack, Hogarty, et al., 2010). In a subsample of 53 of the 58 early-course schizophrenia patients described above, magnetic resonance imaging (MRI) assessments were conducted at baseline, 1 year, and 2 years. Comparing regional volume changes between the two groups at the end of treatment, CET seemed to provide a neuroprotective effect against gray matter loss in temporal lobe structures.

*Integrated Neurocognitive Therapy (INT)*

INT includes both computerized exercises, as well as cognitive-behavioural group sessions and homework assignments meant to promote generalization of training to real-world functioning. Neurocognitive training focuses on processing speed, learning and memory, executive functions, and working memory, whereas social cognitive training focuses on emotion perception, social perception, social schema, and attributional style.

Though INT is a new comer in this area of social cognition intervention, preliminary analyses (Mueller, Schmidt, & Roder, 2011) indicate good treatment tolerability and acceptance of the treatment. Compared to TAU, INT led to improvements in neurocognition, symptoms, functioning, and social cognition, with some indication that treatment gains were maintained or even enhanced at the follow-up assessment. There is also evidence that social cognition and negative symptoms may mediate the relationship between neurocognition and functional outcomes in INT participants (Roder, 2010).

Summary of available social cognition interventions in schizophrenia:

As for as pharmacotherapy is concerned, drugs are yet to be discovered for the treatment of cognitive symptoms including social cognitive deficits. At present psychosocial interventions are the effective available interventions. All the psychosocial interventions have been discussed briefly above and the efficacy/preliminary evidences of various interventions are tabulated below table-3.3.

Apart from psychological interventions, physical exercise including aerobic training had been found to improve social cognition, though the number of studies were just two and the social cognition assessments were not comprehensive(Kimhy et al., 2015) (Firth et al., 2016)

## 3.11 YOGA FOR SOCIAL COGNITION IN SCHIZOPHRENIA

Schizophrenia has also been described in past as split mind/personality. On the other hand, yoga has been defined as *'Citta vṛtti nirodaha'* (controlling the modifications of the mind). In some yoga texts like, Yoga Sutras of Patanjali there are descriptions of experiences like clairaudience and clairvoyance (Iyengar BKS, 2007) which accomplished yoga practitioners cultivate consciously and use for spiritual progress, whereas similar experiences which forms the symptoms of schizophrenia makes the patients socially dysfunctional. Hence, it's likely that the key difference in social functioning and its precursor/predictor – the social cognition could be managed with add-on yoga therapy. In this light, yoga has the potential to be used as an add-on complementary therapy in schizophrenia. Previous studies have demonstrated the efficacy of yoga in schizophrenia for clinical symptoms including some aspects of social cognition like FERD (Jayaram et al., 2013) (R V Behere et al., 2011). To comment on the definite role of yoga for improving symptoms, larger multicentric trials are warranted, as there are only few studies available currently and majority are from India. Hence apparently the evidence available is weak(Broderick, Knowles, Chadwick, & Vancampfort, 2015) and in general there is a trend for yoga studies conducted in India to be positive than in other countries(Cramer, Lauche, Langhorst, & Dobos, 2015)

**Table 3.3 Interventions for Social Cognition training**

| S.No | Author | Study Design | Gender | Patient characteristics | Intervention | Control | Duration of illness | Results |
|---|---|---|---|---|---|---|---|---|
| 1 | Bechi et al. (2012) | RCT( 3 groups; random allocation only for the experimental conditions not for controls) | SRT 63%; SCT 68%; NT 67% | Schizophrenia (n=51); Outpatients. SRT 24, 0 dropout; SCT 28, 1 dropout; NT 24, 2 dropouts | Video based training in AR and ToM; 12 weeks of 1 h session | Social rehabilitation training,CRT 2 one hour sessions per week, for 12 weeks | SRT 15; SCT 14; NT 17 | statistically significant improvement in ToM abilities, but no changes with respect to EP |
| 2 | Bechi et al. (2013) | RCT | ToMI 42%; ACG 54% | Schizophrenia(n=30); 30 outpatients (19 treatment no dropouts; 11 no dropouts) | Theory of Mind Intervention (ToMI); 18 weeks, 1 h sessions twice a week | 18 1 h session twice a week Active control (newspaper discussion group) | ToMI 10.8; ACG 15.4 | significant improvement of ToM abilities among subjects allocated to ToMI compared to ACG |
| 3 | Bechi et al. (2015) | RCT (3 groups) | ToMI 53%; SCT 67%; ACG 53% | Schizophrenia(n=75); 75 outpatients; ToMI 32; SCT 24; ACG 19. Dropouts not Mentioned. | ToMI 18 1 h sessions twice a week; SCT 1 h 12 weeks; plus CRT two 1 h sessions a week | 16 1 h session once a week Active control (newspaper discussion group) | ToMI 16.3; SCT 13.9; ACG 14.94 | SCT and ToMI groups improved significantly in ToM measures, whereas the ACG did not. paranoid and non-paranoid subjects improved significantly after ToMI and SCT, without differences between groups, despite the better performance in basal ToM found among paranoid patients. |
| 4 | Choi and Kwon (2006) | RCT | SCET 52%; Control 58% | Schizophrenia (n=33); Schizoaffective (n=1) Outpatients 17 SCET (7 dropouts); 17 control; 1 Dropouts) | Social Cognition Enhancement Training (SCET) 36 sessions, 1.5 h | Standard psychiatric rehabilitation training (coping skills, medication adherence) | SCET 9.3; Control 13.1 | SCET group significantly improved their performance relative to those in the standard group on one measure of social cognitive ability (PA of WISC-R) |
| 5 | Combs et al. (2007) | Non randomized controlled trial | SCIT 67%; control 90% | Schizophrenia (n=18); 28 forensic inpatients (18 SCIT; 10 control) no information on dropouts | SCIT; 18 h ; 1 session per week | 18 h coping skills group | SCIT 18.4; control 19.7 | compared to the control group, SCIT participants improved on all of the social cognitive measures and showed better selfreported social relationships and fewer aggressive incidents.Change was independent of changes in clinical symptoms |
| 6 | Combs et al. (2008) | RCT (3 groups) | 65.00% | Schizophrenia (n=60); inpatients (20 in each group, no mention of dropouts) | Emotion Perception Intervention (based on attention or monetary incentive) for AR | FEIT only with no training | Not reported | attentional-shaping condition had significantly higher scores on the FEIT at intervention, post-test, and follow-up compared to monetary reinforcement and repeated practice |
| 7 | Corrigan et al. (1995) | RCT | Intervention 45%; control 45% | Schizophrenia (n=46) Inpatient and outpatient; 20 in each group | 1 h session Vigilance plus memory training for social perception (self-instruction, salient cues, repeated practice) | 1 h session Vigilance alone | 59.9 day hospitalised exp.; 61.6 days hospitalised control | subjects in the vigilance-plus-memory condition were able to identify social cues in the videotaped training materials significantly better than subjects in the vigilance-alone condition. Difference was evident in an independent measure of social cue recognition and was present at a 48 h follow-up |

| | | | | | | | | |
|---|---|---|---|---|---|---|---|---|
| 8 | Eack et al. (2009) | RCT | ET 65%; EST 74% | Schizophrenia (n=58); inpatient and outpatient, CET 31, EST 27 (9 dropouts at 1 year, 12 at 2 years) | Cognitive Enhancement Therapy. Two years including 45 1.5 h social cognitive therapy | Enriched Supportive Therapy (EST; incl individual sessions on psychoeducation, relapse prevention) | CET 3.1; EST 3.3 | significant differential effects favoring CET on social cognition, cognitive style, social adjustment, and symptomatology composites during the first year of treatment. After two years, moderate effects (d=.46) were observed favoring CET for enhancing neurocognitive function. Strong differential effects (d>1.00) on social cognition, cognitive style, and social adjustment composites remained at year 2 |
| 9 | Eack et al. (2015) | RCT | CET 68%; TAU 78% | Schizophrenia (n=31); Outpatients with substance misuse. CET 22 (posttreatment 12); TAU 9 (posttreatment 8) | Cognitive Enhancement Therapy. 45 sessions 1.5 h | Treatment as usual | CET 15.2; TAU 11.8 | CET is a feasible and potentially effective treatment for cognitive impairments in patients with schizophrenia who misuse alcohol and/or cannabis. |
| 10 | Garcia et al. (2003) | Non randomized controlled trial | IPTS 82% control 55% | Schizophrenia (n=30); 23 community (IPTS 5: 2 dropouts pre intervention, 6 lost to FU); 7 control (1 before test, 2 lost to FU) | Integrated Psychological Therapy for Schizophrenia Patients (IPTS) | No training condition | IPTS 21; control 15 | instrument has been sensitive to changes in the pre-treatment and post-treatment measures, showing that schizophrenics patients have improved their ability to perceive and to interpret reality in a more adequate way. |
| 11 | Gil Sanz et al. (2009) | RCT | PECS 57%; control 43% | Schizophrenia (n=14); 14 community patients (PECS 7; control 7) no information on dropouts | Social Cognition Training Program (PECS) | nclear but difference is that control group only received ER training, not SP | PECS 13.4; control 20.6 | improvement in social perception and interpretation in the experimental group, in comparison with the control group, but not in emotion recognition. No significant correlations were obtained between social cognition training and other variables tested. |
| 12 | Gil-Sanz et al. (2014) | RCT | PECS 40%; control 66% | Schizophrenia (n=83); 83 community patients (PECS 44; control 39) no information on dropouts | Social Cognition Training Program (PECS) | Attention and memory | PECS 12; control 16 | experimental group showed a higher performance compared to patients in the control task group in the Hinting Task Test and in the emotion recognition of sadness, anger, fear, and disgust |
| 13 | Gohar, Hamdi, El Ray, Horan and Green (2013) | RCT | SCST 72%; control 90% | Schizophrenia (n=42); outpatients (SCST 22; Control 20. No dropouts) | Social Cognitive Skills Training.2 sessions per week for 8 weeks | Skills Training Control Group. 16 sessions | SCST 21.6; control 22.5 | SCST group demonstrated significant treatment effects on total emotional intelligence scores, as well as the sub-areas of Identifying Emotions and Managing Emotions , compared with those in the control condition. There were no treatment benefits for neurocognition for either condition, and both interventions were well-tolerated by patients |

| | | | | | | | | |
|---|---|---|---|---|---|---|---|---|
| 14 | Hasson-Ohayon et al. (2014) | RCT | 69.00% | Schizophrenia (n=55) community patients (SCIT-34, control-21); no drop cuts | SCIT, plus social mentoring 8 weeks, one hour sessions | Social mentoring, Three times per week, 1 h | Not reported | preliminary evidence that SCIT plus social mentoring improves social cognition and functioning among persons with severe mental illness who are living in the community |
| 15 | Habel et al. (2010) | RCT | 100% | Schizophrenia(n=30 ) 30 inpatient and outpatient (10 treatment group 4 dropouts; 10 TAU 2 dropouts; | 12 sessions of 45 mins Training in Affect Recognition (TAR) | Treatment as usual (no additional information); Healthy controls | Not reported | patients differentially impaired in the identification of the emotional aspects of facial expressions (but not age discrimination) compared to healthy participants. increased number of correct identifications was observed in trained patients only. an increase in activation was noted in the left middle and superior occipital lobe, the right inferior and superior parietal cortex, and the inferior frontal cortex bilaterally in TAR patients compared to the TAU group. These activation changes in TAR patients correlated with their behavioral improvement, |
| 16 | Horan et al. (2009) | RCT | SCT 87%; Control 100% | Schizophrenia (n=34) (SCIT 15 2 dropouts; Control 16 1 dropout) | Social Cognitive Training; 12 1 h once a week | Active control group 12 1 h once a week; illness management and relapse prevention skills training | SCT 20.2; control 18.0 | individuals who received the social cognitive intervention demonstrated significant improvements in facial affect perception, one of the four targeted social cognitive domains. These improvements were not attributable to changes in neurocognitive functioning or clinical symptoms. |
| 17 | Horan et al. (2011) | RCT | SCST 93.8%; NR 89.5%, ST 78.9%; Hybrid 92.9% | 68 patients ( (48 schizophrenia,13 schizoaffective,7 psychosis NOS) (SCST 16, 3 dropouts; NR 19, 5 dropouts; Hybrid 14 (7 dropouts) | Social Cognitive Skills Training;24 sessions, Neurocognitive remediation; Hybrid combination. | ST – standard illness management training. Matched for contact time. | SCST 19.7 yrs.; NR 22.7 yrs.; ST 24.1 yrs.; Hybrid 23.4 yrs | The SCST group demonstrated greater improvements over time than comparison groups in the social cognitive domain of emotional processing, including improvement on measures of facial affect perception and emotion management. There were no differential benefits among treatment conditions on neurocognitive or clinical symptom changes over time. |
| 18 | Kayser et al. (2006) | RCT | Intervention 60%; control 84% | Schizophrenia (n=14) (13 outpatients, 1 being discharged) (8 exp.; 6 control) dropouts not reported | 2 one hour training sessions, Video clips showing social interactions, with training in theory of mind | Treatment as usual | Intervention 12.3; control 11.5 | patients showed less disorganisation signs on the second evaluation when compared to the first (there seems to be a possible improvement of the participants' communication disorders and their ability to attribute intentions to others) |

| | | | | | | | | |
|---|---|---|---|---|---|---|---|---|
| 19 | Mazza et al. (2010) | RCT | 59% | Schizophrenia (n=33) ETIT group 17; control group 16. 0 dropouts | Two days a week, 12 weeks 50 mins. Emotion and ToM Imitation Training (ETIT) | Problem solving group | Intervention 6.3; control 6.5 | ETIT participants improved on every social cognitive measure and showed better social functioning at posttest than controls . Improvement in social cognition, in particular in emotion recognition, is also supported by ERP responses: we recorded an increase in electroactivity of medio-frontal areas only after ETIT treatment. |
| 20 | Penn and Combs (2000) | RCT (4 groups) | 58% | Schizophrenia (n=40) (10; 12; 9; 9 group split) dropout info not reported | Reinforcement, facial feedback and combination targeting FAR. | Repeated practice condition with no feedback | 17.1 | all groups of subjects, with the exception of those in the repeated practice group, improved in their ability to identify facial affect, with these effects showing some stability over time. There was limited evidence of these effects generalizing to the test of facial affect discrimination. |
| 21 | Popova et al. (2014) | RCT( 3 groups) | 66% | Schizophrenia (n=57) FAT 29, 10 dropouts; TAU 24, 5 dropouts); CE 27, 8 dropouts | FAT consisted of training in affect recognition and working memory. 20 daily 1 h sessions over 4 weeks | CE standardised program of cognitive training, and treatment as usual | Not reported | alpha power increase during the dynamic facial affect recognition task was larger after affect training than after treatment-as-usual, though similar to that after targeted perceptual–cognitive training. Alpha power modulation was unrelated to general neuropsychological test performance, and it improved in all group |
| 22 | Roberts et al. (2014) | RCT | SCIT 67% TAU; 67% | Schizophrenian (n=66) (SCIT 33, 2 drop outs; TAU 33, 1 dropout) | 20–24 Weekly hour long sessions of SCIT | TAU | SCIT 23; TAU 23 | SCIT may improve social functioning, negative symptoms, and possibly hostile attributional bias. Post-hoc analyses suggest a dose– response effect. |
| 23 | Roncone et al. (2004) | RCT | Intervention 60%; control 70% | Schizophrenia (n=20) (10 exp.; 10 control) dropouts not mentioned | Metacognitive Intervention Programme; 22 h of training to change social cognitive structure | Medication and supportive psychotherapy "where needed" | Intervention 16.9; control 11.1 | Social cognition, neurocognition, clinical variables, and community functioning improved significantly following metacognitive training based rehabilitation |
| 24 | Russell et al. (2008) | RCT | Intervention 65%; 71% control | Schizophrenia (n=40) (26 in exp. groups, 13 in control 1 dropout in ctrl) | METT | Repeated exposure | Intervention 21.6; control 23.6 | first evidence that improvements in emotion recognition following METT training are associated with changes in visual attention to the feature areas of emotional faces |

| | | | | | | | | |
|---|---|---|---|---|---|---|---|---|
| 25 | Sachs et al. (2012) | RCT | TAR 60%; TAU 40% | Schizophrenia (n=40) inpatients and outpatients (TAR 20, 0 dropouts; control 18, 2 dropouts) | 12 sessions over 6 weeks; Training in Affect Recognition | 12 sessions over 6 weeks Treatment as usual | TAR 24.3; TAU 24.3 | TAR group achieved significant improvements in facial affect recognition, in particular in recognizing sad faces and, in addition, in the quality of life domain social relationship. TAR training contributes to enhancing some aspects of cognitive functioning and negative symptoms. improvements in facial affect recognition and quality of life were independent of changes in clinical symptoms and general cognitive functions. |
| 26 | Tas et al. (2012) | RCT | F-SCIT 57.9%; SS 46.2% | Schizophrenia (n=49) outpatients (F-SCIT 19, 3 dropouts; SS 26, 1 dropout) | 14 weeks; based on SCIT program | 14 weeks; Social Stimulation (SS) | F-SCIT 12.6; SS 11.9 | Patients who received FSCIT significantly improved in quality of life, social functioning and social cognition, whereas the SS group worsened in nearly all outcome variables. Family-assisted SCIT is effective in improving quality of life, social functioning and social cognition |
| 27 | Taylor et al. (2015) | RCT | 100% (single sex ward) | Schizophrenia (n=45) forensic inpatients (SCIT 21, 5 dropouts; TAU 15 4 dropouts) | 16 sessions, twice a week for 45 min. Based on SCIT | TAU | SCIT 25,2; TAU 22.3 | SCIT group showed a significant improvement in facial affect recognition compared to TAU |
| 28 | van der Gaag et al. (2002) | RCT | Intervention 62%; control 66% | Schizophrenia (n=42) inpatients (21 per group, 3 dropouts | 22 sessions, training on perception; reasoning, emotion perception and social situations | Treatment same as experimental group, but leisure activities substituted for intervention | Not reported | cognitive training program improved emotion perception, with some evidence of generalization to measures of executive functioning; other areas of neurocognitive functioning were largely unaffected |
| 29 | Veltro et al. (2011) | RCT | Not reported | Schizophrenia (n=24) outpatients | 24 sessions, 90 min Cognitive Emotional Rehabilitation (REC) | 24 sessions, 90 min Problem solving training (PST) | REC 14.2; PST 11.9 | both training methods(REC & PST) were found to be effective in psychopathological measures and in social functioning. On cognitive function improvements were specific to the rehabilitative approach. PST are mainly improved capacities for planning and memory, while the REC improved measures such as social cognition Theory of mind and emotion recognition |
| 30 | Wang et al. (2013) | RCT | SCIT 54.5%, TAU 47.1% | Schizophrenia (n=43) outpatients (SCIT 22, 0 dropouts; Control 21, 4 dropouts) | 20 weeks based on SCIT | Treatment as usual | Not reported | Patients in SCIT group showed a significant improvement in the domains of emotion perception, theory of mind, attributional style, and social functioning compared to those in waiting-list group. |

| | | | | | | | | |
|---|---|---|---|---|---|---|---|---|
| 31 | Wolwer et al. (2005) | RCT (3 groups) | TAR 90%; CRT 58%; control 84% | Schizophrenia (n=77) inpatients & outpatients TAR 28; CRT 24; 25 TAU (24 dropouts) | 12 sessions TAR facial affect recognition; 12 sessions CRT neurocognition | TAU | Number of previous hospitalisations (TAR 4.8; CR T 6.2; TAU 3.3) | Patients under TAR significantly improved in facial affect recognition, with recognition performance after training; Patients under CRT and those without special training (TAU) did not improve in affect recognition, though patients under CRT improved in verbal memory functions |
| 32 | Wolwer and Frommann (2011) | RCT | 68% | Schizophrenia (n=38) inpatients (TAR 20, 5 dropouts; CRT 18, 3 drops outs) | TAR facial affect recognition; 12 sessions 45–60 min | CRT neurocognition;12 sessions 45–60 min | 7 first episode, 13 2–4 episodes, 13 had 5 or more | Intentionto-treat analyses found significantly larger pre–post improvements with TAR than with CRT in prosodic affect recognition, ToM, and social competence and a trend effect in global social functioning. |

# Chapter 4.0

# AIMS & OBJECTIVES

# 4.0 AIMS & OBJECTIVES

## 4.1 AIM

To study the effect of yoga based intervention on social cognition in patients with schizophrenia.

## 4.2 OBJECTIVES

***Primary objective***

1. To study the effect of add-on yoga therapy on Social Cognition measures (composite score of SOCRATIS and TRENDS)

***Secondary objective***

1. To study the effect of add-on yoga therapy on Mirror Neuron Activity (MNA) using functional Near Infrared Spectroscopy (fNIRS) in patients with schizophrenia.

## 4.3 RESEARCH QUESTION

1. Can add-on yoga therapy improve social cognition scores measured by SOCRATIS and TRENDs in patients with schizophrenia?

2) Can add-on yoga therapy enhance MNA measured by fNIRS in patients with schizophrenia

## 4.4 RESEARCH HYPOTHESES

***Alternate hypothesis***

$H_a1$: Add-on Yoga therapy will enhance SOCRATIS & TRENDS scores in patients with schizophrenia.

$H_a2$: Add-on yoga therapy will enhance MNA measured by fNIRS in patients with schizophrenia

***Null Hypotheses***

$H_01$: Add-on Yoga therapy will not enhance SOCRATIS & TRENDS scores in patients with schizophrenia

H02: Add-on yoga therapy will enhance MNA measured by fNIRS in patients with schizophrenia

## 4.5 RATIONALE OF THE STUDY

Inspite of the availability of various psychosocial interventions, still the translation of research evidence into clinical utility is highly questionable. For example, one of the interventions- Cognitive Enhancement Therapy(CET) has a robust evidence for social cognition improvement including the neurocognition and functioning level. But its application in real world scenario is doubtful as it is highly resource intensive. Similar is the issue with majority of available psychosocial interventions, especially in countries like India, where there is a huge imbalance in clinician/therapist and patient ratio. Also, the suitability of the available interventions in Indian population are yet to be investigated, in the context of cultural differences.

Hence exploring other alternative therapies for cognitive deficit in schizophrenia is the need of the hour. Yoga has been in use widely for various lifestyle disorders including mental health conditions like depression, anxiety and pain disorders. Yoga has been found to improve cognition in healthy population (Gothe & McAuley, 2015) and in some non-psychiatric conditions (Velikonja, Čurić, Ožura, & Jazbec, 2010) (Chattha R, Nagarathna R, Padmalatha V, 2008). Utility of yoga for cognition in mental health disorders is an area that needs exploration (Hariprasad et al., 2013). Earlier studies have looked into Facial Emotion Recognition Deficit (FERD) and oxytocin levels with yoga intervention in schizophrenia (Jayaram et al., 2013) (R V Behere et al., 2011), but a comprehensive investigation of social cognition with yoga intervention in schizophrenia has not been done earlier.

# Chapter 5.0
# METHODS

# 5.0 METHODS

## 5.1 SETTING

The study was conducted at National Institute of Mental Health & Neuro Sciences (NIMHANS) in collaboration with S-VYASA Yoga University.

Ethical Clearance:

Study was approved by the Ethics Committee of both the institutions.

Eligible and willing subjects were explained about the nature of the trial including possible adverse effects in the language understandable to them. Subjects were explained about their equal chance in falling to either yoga therapy or waitlist control group. They were also explained about their right to withdraw from the trial at any point of time if they wished not to continue, without any impact on their regular treatment by the treating team. All the subjects were recruited with written informed consent.

Copy of informed consent and ethics committee approval letter is attached in the appendix.

## 5.2 STUDY DESIGN

Randomized controlled trial

## 5.3 SELECTION OF SUBJECTS

***Inclusion criteria***

1. Diagnosis of schizophrenia (DSM-5) (American Psychiatric Association, 2013b)
2. CGI-S Score $\geq$3 (Clinical Global Impression - Severity) (Guy W, 2000).Schizophrenia patients stabilized with antipsychotic medication for minimum 4-6 weeks.
3. Age range: 18-45years
4. Either sex
5. Written informed consent

***Exclusion criteria***

1. Features suggestive of risk of harm to self (example-suicidal risk) or others (example-aggression)

2. Need for Electroconvulsive therapy/given ECT in last three months.
3. Co-morbid substance dependence in the past 6 months or substance abuse in the past 1 month as per DSM 5, except nicotine.
4. Significant neurological disorder like seizure disorder, recent head injury, etc. evaluated by detailed neurologic examination.
5. Lifetime history of significant head injury
6. Pregnancy or postpartum (<6 weeks after delivery)

The demographic and clinical information (history of present illness as well as any other medical illness, family & personal history) regarding the patients was collected using structured proforma.
Diagnosis of schizophrenia was made as per DSM- 5 by a psychiatry resident and confirmed using Mini-International Neuro psychiatric Interview (M.I.N.I.) (Sheehan et al., 1998) Psychopathology was assessed using structured assessment scales.

## 5.4 SAMPLE SIZE CALCULATION

Sample size was calculated based on the effect size (d=1.1) for the Facial Emotion Recognition task, from a previous study (Jayaram et al., 2013) .Sample size required to detect a significant difference in the variable of interest with a power of .80, allowing for 5% type I error, was 32 (16 in each arm). Considering the drop out of 16% in previous studies, sample size was rounded to 40 (20 in each arm)

## 5.5 SUBJECTS RECRUITMENT & RANDOMIZATION

Schizophrenia patients attending services at psychiatry department (outpatients=29; inpatients=11) of NIMHANS, were assessed for eligibility by a psychiatry resident and the diagnosis was confirmed using Mini-International Neuro Psychiatric Interview (MINI). With written informed consent, patients who were stabilized on antipsychotics for at least 6 weeks and were co-operative for yoga practices were recruited. Out of 478 screened subjects, 339 were eligible for study and 40 eligible subjects agreed for participation in the study. The data was collected from March 2016 to July 2017. Random assignment of eligible and willing subjects to Yoga Therapy Group(YT) or Waitlist Control (WL) was done by the research scholar with Sequentially Numbered Opaque Sealed Envelope(SNOSE) method. Computer generated random numbers were used for treatment assignment. Random numbers were generated by a scientific officer who was not involved in assessment or recruitment of the subjects.

## 5.6 INTERVENTION

### *Yoga module validation*

We began by reviewing the classical and contemporary yoga related texts to develop the content of the module. Texts on *Patanjali yoga sutras*, *Hatha yoga pradipika*, *Shiva samhita*, *Gerhanda samhita*, *Hatharatnavali*, *Bhagavad gita*, *Upanishads* and *Yoga vasistha* were reviewed (Iyengar BKS, 2007) (Muktibodhananda, 1998) (Pancham Singh & Rai Bahadur Srisa Chandra Vasu, 2009) (Mahadevan TMP, 2010)(Sri Janananda Bharati, 1982) (Chinmaya International Foundation, 2012).

Practices that could potentially target positive, negative, and cognitive symptoms as well as medication-related side-effects were searched from classical and contemporary literature. Although the practices included were based on traditional texts, these do not give exact symptom-based guidelines for practices; yoga is a science meant for achieving liberation and not for therapy. Hence the components of the module have been selected by approximating descriptions of mental and physical benefits of specific yoga practices with the symptom dimensions of schizophrenia. Practices which may be difficult to teach and practice for patients with schizophrenia and those that are contraindicated in common disorders like hypertension, cardiovascular diseases, etc. were excluded. Likewise, practices that pose difficulty to objectively verify, were not chosen. To suit the patients' needs, like use of wall support some practices were modified. The yoga module that was designed is composed of slow movements with breathing awareness, loosening exercises including *surya namaskara*, *asanas*, *pranayama*, *Om japa* and relaxation. The duration of the yoga module is approximately one hour.

*Validation process*

The designed yoga module was sent along with three case vignettes of adults with symptoms of schizophrenia to 30 Yoga experts, of whom 10 experts responded with their scores and comments. The experts rated the usefulness of the practices in the module on a scale of 1-5 (1- not at all useful; 2- little useful; 3- moderately useful; 4- very much useful; 5-extremely useful). Content Validity Ratio (CVR) for suitability of items and Intra Class Correlation (ICC) coefficient for inter rater reliability were calculated. Dichotomous (yes/no) and qualitative responses were also obtained from the experts to determine the appropriateness of duration of each yoga session and the whole yoga training programme. Details of the yoga module is given below (table-5.1) and discussed in detail in earlier publication (Govindaraj, Varambally, Sharma, & Gangadhar, 2016).

Validated Yoga module was administered (Subject performing yoga, Figure-5.1) to the Yoga group for 60 min, 4-5 sessions per week, with a total of 20 sessions to be completed within 6 weeks. Maximum 3 subjects were taught together in a session. Majority of the subjects finished 20 sessions in 6 weeks. Few subjects finished in 4 weeks. Waitlist participants were offered Yoga after 6 weeks.

**Table-5.1 Yoga module**

| S.No | Practice | Duration |
|---|---|---|
| | Loosening Exercises | |
| 1 | Jogging | 1min 45 sec |
| 2 | Mukha Dhouti | 30 sec |
| 3 | Twisting | 1 min |
| 4 | Hand stretch breathing | 1 min |
| 5 | Forward & Backward bending | 1 min |
| 6 | Tiger breathing | 1 min |
| 7 | Sideward bending | 1 min |
| 8 | Shashankasana breathing | 1 min |

| | | |
|---|---|---|
| 9 | Surya namaskar (12 rounds) | 10-15min |
| | Yogasana | |
| 1 | Vakrasana | 1 min |
| 2 | Ustrasana | 1 min |
| 3 | Bhujangasana | 1 min |
| 4 | Shalabhasana | 1 min |
| 5 | Dhanurasana | 1 min |
| 6 | Vipreetakarani | 3 min |
| 7 | Matsyasana | 1 min |
| | Pranayama | |
| 1 | Bhastrika | 2.5 min |
| 2 | Nadishuddhi | 3 min |
| | Chanting Meditation/Relaxation | |
| 1 | Nadhanusandhana(A,U,M & AUM Chanting) | 10 min |
| 2 | Quick Relaxation Technique | 4 min |
| | | |
| | Total Duration | 50-60 min |
| | | |

## 5.7 ASSESSMENTS

A trained yoga therapist gave the yoga intervention to subjects. A Psychiatry resident did the clinical assessments and was blind to the treatment allocation. Clinical assessments (positive symptoms, negative symptoms and social disability/functioning) which are subjective were assessed by a blind assessor (Psychiatry resident) and the social cognition assessment which is a computer based objective test (less prone to bias), was done by non-blinded research scholar.

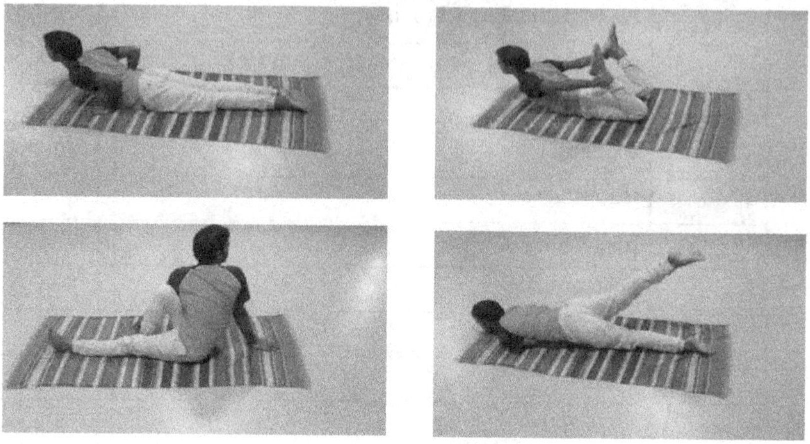

**Fig-5.1 Subject performing Yoga (with subject's consent)**

All the assessments were done at the baseline and at the end of 20 sessions of Yoga training. Timeline and the details of assessment variables are as follows,

**Table-5.2 Assessment details and timeline**

| S.no | Variables | Baseline | $4^{th}$ week/end of 20 sessions yoga |
|---|---|---|---|
| 1 | SOCRATIS | + | + |
| 2 | TRENDS | + | + |
| 3 | MNA-fNIRS | + | + |
| 4 | SANS & SAPS | + | + |
| 5 | GSDS-II | + | + |
| 6 | CGI | + | + |
| 7 | B-CATS | + | + |

***Intake Proforma***

A structured proforma was used to collect the details of socio-demographic and clinical variables including age-at-onset, type of onset, and duration of illness

***Mini-International Neuropsychiatric Interview (M.I.N.I.)***

MINI is a short structured diagnostic interview for DSM-IV-TR and ICD-10 psychiatric disorders.

***Social Cognition Rating Tool in Indian Setting (SOCRATIS)***

SOCRATIS is a tool, which was validated, in the Indian socio-cultural context to assess social cognition in schizophrenia patients. It assesses theory of mind (first order, second order and faux pas), attribution styles (32 point questionnaire) and social perception [SoCueReTI -Social Cue Recognition Test-Indian setting].

Consistent with expert committee recommendations (Green et al., 2008) , we selected 4 out of the 5 recommended social cognition domains, namely, Theory of Mind (ToM), emotion processing, social perception, and attributional bias. ToM, social perception and attributional bias will be assessed using the Social Cognition Rating Tools in Indian Setting (SOCRATIS). Emotion processing will be assessed using the Tool for Recognition of Emotions in Neuropsychiatric DisorderS (TRENDS) (Rishikesh V Behere et al., 2008).

SOCRATIS and TRENDS have undergone cultural adaptation (e.g., use of native names, attire, and actors) and translational procedures (e.g., using conceptual, rather than literal, translations in two Indian languages) to modify the tasks to the Indian cultural setting, without disturbing the actual social cognition constructs that they were meant to test. The content validity, in terms of fidelity to the original construct and cultural appropriateness of these tasks has been found to be satisfactory. When tested on bilinguals, there was good concurrence of their performance in the original and the modified tasks (concurrent validity). These procedures and their validation have been described in further detail in previous studies.

To avoid learning effect, each domain in SOCRATIS was divided equally into two parts. One part was used at the baseline and the second part was used at the end of 20 sessions of Yoga training.

*Theory of mind*

Tasks included two each of 1st order [based on Sally-Anne (Wimmer & Perner, 1983) and Smarties tasks], 2nd order false belief picture stories [based on ice-cream van (Perner & Wimmer, 1985) and missing cookies (Stone, Baron-

Cohen, & Knight, 1998) tasks], two metaphor–irony stories [adapted from (Drury, Robinson, & Birchwood, 1998)] and ten faux pas recognition stories [based on the faux pas recognition test(Stone et al., 1998)]. These story-based tasks examine the ability at different complexity levels to 'meta-represent' mental states of others (e.g., Suresh thinks that Rani will go to the temple area to buy the ice-cream because she has not seen the ice-cream man go towards the school).

Following are the different ToM tasks used in SOCRATIS

**Table-5.3 ToM Assessment tasks**

| Domain | Task |
|---|---|
| First order ToM | Shanti Ravi task & Sweet box task (modified from Sally-Anne task & smarties task) |
| Second order ToM | Ice-cream man task & Hidden bananas task (modified from ice-cream van task & Missing cookies task) |
| Metaphor-Irony | Metaphor-Irony stories (modified from Metaphor-Irony stories) |
| Faux pas | Faux pas recognition test (modified from Faux pas recognition test) |

*Attributional bias*

This was assessed using a 32-point questionnaire where subjects were required to make causal attributions for positive and negative social events, adapted from the Internal, Personal, and Situational Attributions Questionnaire (Kinderman & Bentall, 1996)

*Social perception*

A set of 18 true/false questions were asked on social (e.g., Ali asked many questions about the movie because he was trying to impress Sunil) and non-social cues (e.g., Harish and Lakshmi were looking over a book together) after showing the subjects four each of low and high emotion videos depicting a social interaction. This test was adapted from the social cue recognition test (Corrigan & Green, 1993a).

As mentioned above, both SOCRATIS and TRENDS have been validated in the Indian cultural setting. Their psychometric properties (content, concurrent and known-groups validity, internal consistency and external validity) have been found to be satisfactory. Each test, except attributional bias, provides an index of the respective test performance, which is equivalent to the score of an individual on the test divided by the maximum score possible. We consider metaphor and irony detection as 1st and 2nd order ToM respectively. Faux pas recognition is often described as a higher order ToM ability (Brüne, 2005)

*Tool for Recognition of Emotions in Neuropsychiatric DisorderS (TRENDS)*

This is a tool validated for use in the Indian population (Rishikesh V Behere et al., 2008), which captures the full range and nature of emotional expressions akin to real life situations and can be utilized for behavioural and functional imaging studies in Indian patients. It takes into account variations of age and sex on emotional expressions and is a culture-sensitive tool. This is a culturally sensitive, ecologically valid tool, consisting of 52 static (still) and 28 dynamic (video clip) images (i.e. totally 80 images) of six basic emotions – happy, sad, fear, anger, surprise, disgust, and a neutral expression emoted by four experienced actors (one young man, one young woman, one older man, and one older woman).

Scale for Assessment of Negative Symptoms (SANS) & Scale for Assessment of Positive Symptoms SAPS: (Andreasen, 1984a) (Andreasen, 1984b)
The SANS is a 25-item scale designed to assess the negative symptom complex in five domains including alogia, affective flattening, avolition-apathy, anhedonia-asociality and attention. The SAPS is a 34-item scale designed to assess positive symptoms of schizophrenia in four domains of hallucinations, delusions, bizarre behavior and formal thought disorder. Ratings were done based on clinical interview, direct observation and any additional sources of information. The scale is on 0-5 spectrum (0=not present, 5=severe). It takes around 15-20 minutes to administer the scale

***Groningen Social Disabilities Schedule (GSDS-II)***

The Groningen Social Disabilities Schedule (Wiersma, DeJong, & Ormel, 1988), which is a semi-structured, culture-neutral interview, based on the WHO Disability Assessment Schedule-II was employed for assessment of socio-occupational functioning of patients.

***Clinical Global Impression (CGI)***

CGI-S (severity) was used at the baseline for assessing severity of the illness and CGI-I (Improvement) was used at the end of one month of intervention (Guy W, 2000).

***Brief Cognitive Assessment Tool for Schizophrenia (B-CATS)***

B-CATS comprises of three tasks i.e., Digit Symbol-Coding, Semantic Fluency, and Trail Making Test-B. Its reliability and Validity have been well established. It is easy to administer and takes less than 15 minutes to complete the assessment (Hurford, Marder, Keefe, Reise, & Bilder, 2011).

Clinical assessments (SANS, SAPS, GSDS & CGI) were done by psychiatry resident, who was blind to the treatment allocation. Social Cognition including MNA measured by fNIRS and neuropsychological tests (B-CATS) were done by the research scholar. Yoga Performance by the subjects were monitored by trained yoga therapist. Blinding of the research scholar was not possible as yoga was taught to the subjects by the research scholar. However, the social cognition assessment done by research scholar is a computer based objective test and is not prone to bias unlike the clinical scales.

**Functional Near Infra-Red Spectroscopy (fNIRS) methods**

Optical data was acquired with a continuous wave fNIRS system [2 wavelengths (760nm & 850nm), 8 sources, 4 detectors, sampling frequency 6.25-Hz) (NIRScout, NIRx Medical Technologies, LLC, CA, USA). Based on 10-20 system, the optodes were placed with the help of a tight-fitting cap in a band like configuration covering locations corresponding left ventral premotor cortex relevant for mirror neuron activity (Fig-5.2). The average distance between optodes was about 3cm. fNIRS data was acquired during the paradigm for mirror neuronal activation (paradigm details as described below).

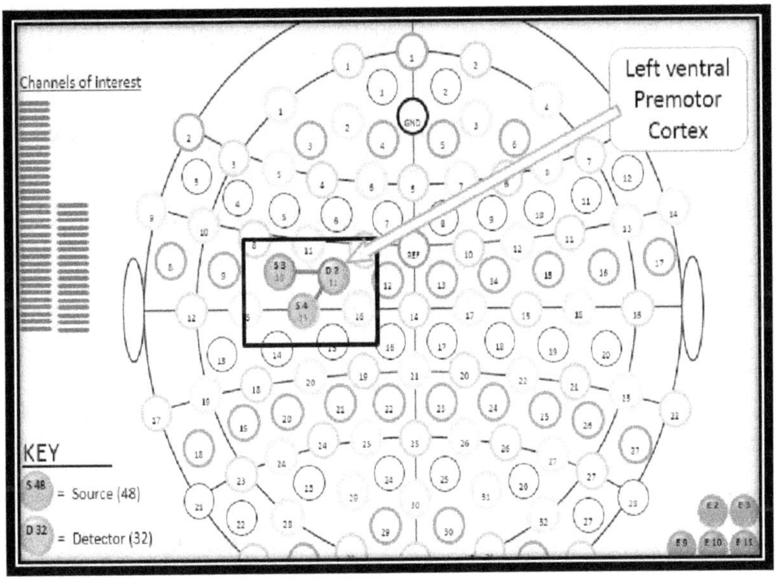


**Figure-5.2 Probe Geometry for Left Ventral Premotor Cortex**

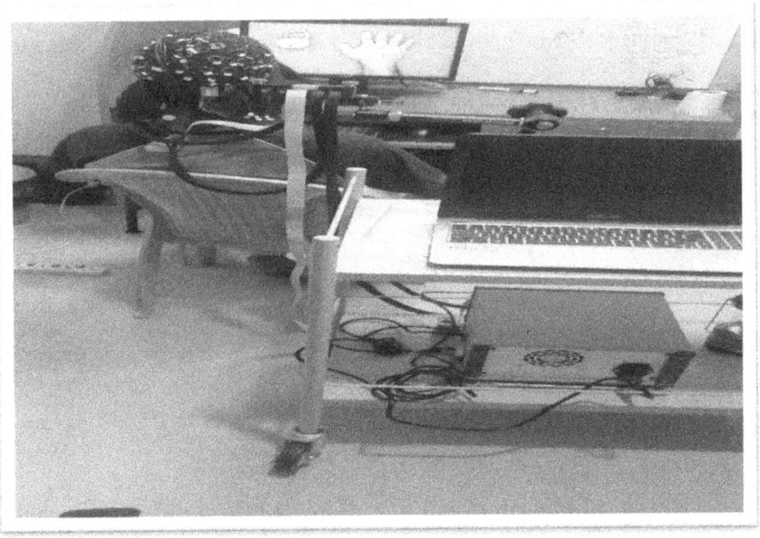

**Figure-5.3 Subject undergoing MNA task with fNIRS**

Paradigm used for eliciting MNA is as follows,

After recording the baseline BOLD signal for 30 seconds, the subjects were given the following tasks while continuing the fNIRS experiment.

1. Static image/Resting state (60 seconds): The subjects were asked to observe a still image of a hand and a lock displayed on the monitor. See Fig-5.4

2a. Action observation (motor paradigm) (60 seconds): The subjects were asked to observe a video, which depicts the experimenter's hand, holding a key in lateral pinch grip (grasping objects between the side of the index finger and the thumb) to perform locking/unlocking actions. This action requires contraction of the FDI to abduct the index finger. See Fig-5.4

2b. Action observation (emotionally embedded motor paradigm) (90 seconds): In this condition, subjects were asked to observe a video of the emotionally embedded motor action that was developed in the earlier studies. An emotional context was shown in the video related to the action to be observed by the subjects (e.g., a person is desperately trying to open a jammed lock of a door to a room inside which someone is trapped). This action requires contraction of the FDI muscle of the person in the video to abduct the index finger while holding the key for unlocking. This paradigm was shown to give more consistent mirror neuron activation and has shown to enhance difference in MNA between healthy individuals and those with psychiatric disorders including schizophrenia (Bagewadi, Mehta, Thirthalli, & Gangadhar, 2014).

3. Action execution (60 seconds): Subjects were asked to execute the action of locking/unlocking with the hand holding a key in lateral pinch grip (grasping objects between the side of the index finger and the thumb)

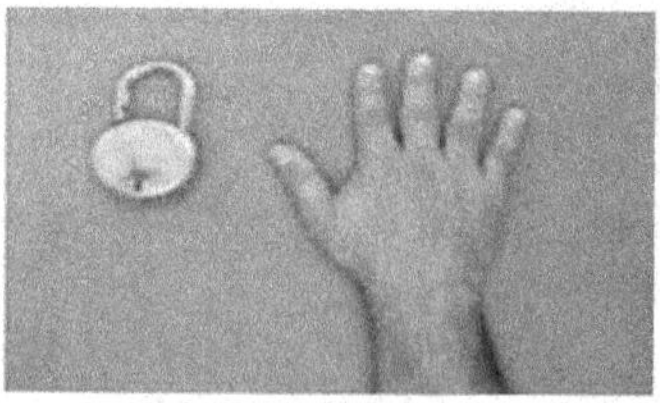

Static Image

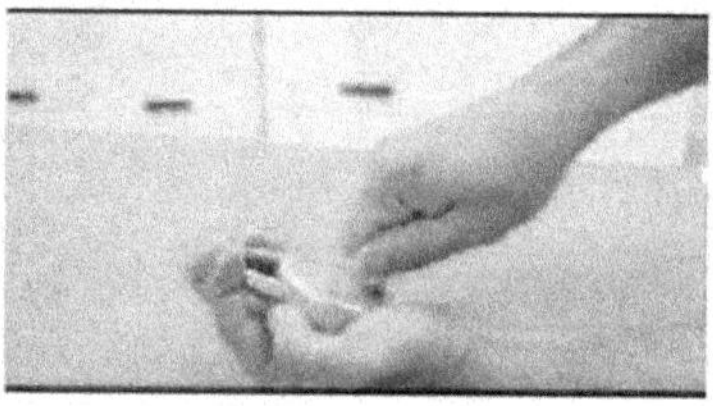

Dynamic Action

**Fig-5.4 MNA paradigms**

The sequence of displaying these experimental states to each subject were randomized. In order to guarantee optimal attention allocation during the fNIRS experiments, subjects were instructed to pay attention to all the stimuli throughout the experiment.

Mirror neuron Activity was deduced by the difference in BOLD signal between a) action execution and resting state and b) action observation and resting state. An increment in BOLD (Blood Oxygen Level Dependant)-signal from premotor and motor cortices during action observation/execution relative to rest states was obtained a measure of putative MNA.

# Chapter 6.0

# DATA EXTRACTION & ANALYSIS

# 6.0 DATA EXTRACTION & ANALYSIS

## 6.1 NIRS DATA

Data was processed using the NIRS LAB software for topographical analysis and GLM computations on NIRS time series data (https://www.nitrc.org/projects/fnirs_downstate/)

## 6.2 CLINICAL, SOCIAL COGNITION AND NEUROPSYCHOLOGICAL ASSESSMENTS

Data collected in assessment forms were screened for completeness and entered in excel sheet. Data was also screened for outliers and then analyzed using SPSS version 24. Chi square test was applied for categorical variables and t test/RMANOVA/Wilcoxon sign rank tests is/are applied for numerical variables.

# Chapter 7.0
# RESULTS

# 7.0 RESULTS

The trial profile is depicted in CONSORT flowchart in Fig-7.1.

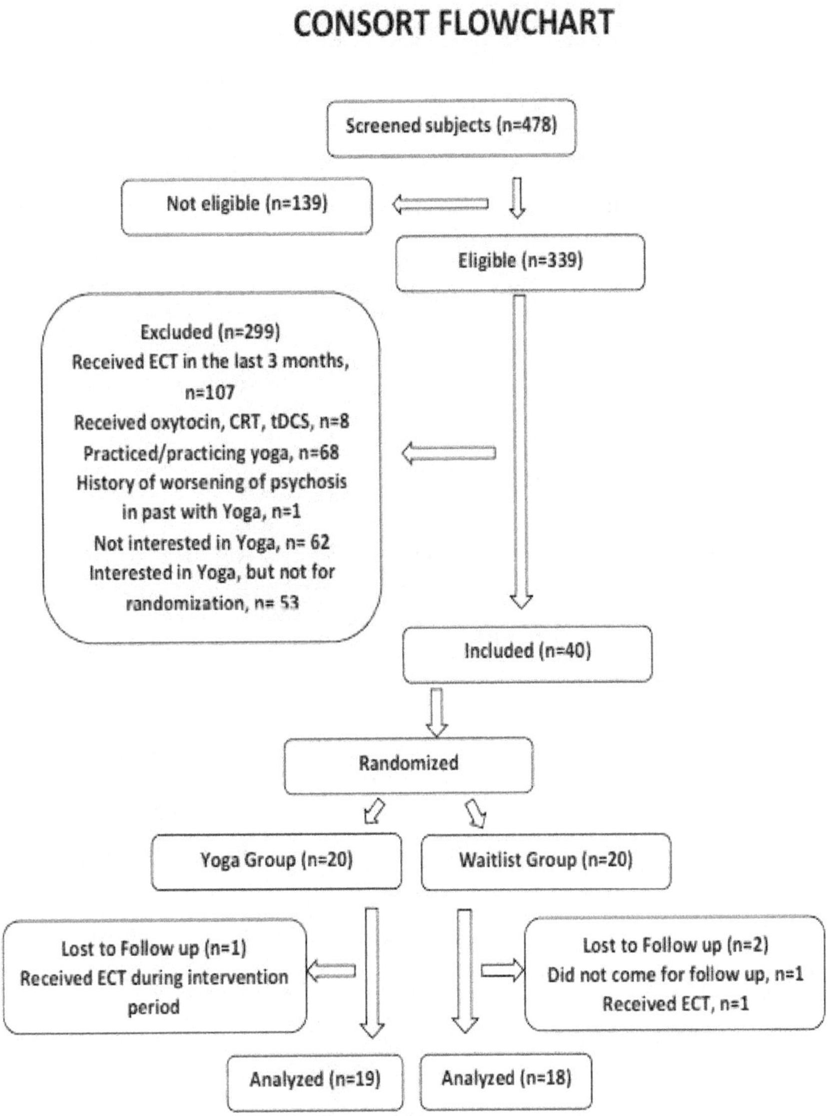


**Figure -7.1 Trial profile**

Note: ECT-Electroconvulsive therapy; tDCS-transcranial Direct Current Stimulation; CRT- Cognitive Remediation Therapy

Outpatients and inpatients of psychiatry department at NIMHANS were screened for eligibility. Out of the 478 subjects screened, 339 were found to be eligible. From the eligible subjects, 299 were excluded for various reasons (107 patients received ECT in the last 3 months; 8 subjects received oxytocin/tDCS-transcranial Direct Current Stimulation/CRT-Cognitive Remediation Therapy; 68 subjects were practicing yoga already; 62 subjects had no interest in practicing yoga; 53 subjects wanted yoga immediately and did not opt for randomization and one subject had worsening of psychosis with Sudarshan Kriya Yoga in the past). Forty subjects were recruited finally and randomized to yoga group (20) and waitlist group (20). Two subjects dropped in the waitlist group (one received ECT; one did not turn for follow up). In the yoga group one subject dropped (received ECT during the intervention period). Thirty-seven subjects were available for the final analysis (19-yoga group & 18 Waitlist group)

## 7.1 BASELINE AND DEMOGRAPHIC DATA (Table -7.1)

Subjects were compared for age, sex, marital status, years of education, duration of illness, illness severity, medication dosage (CPZ equivalents), clinical symptoms and social and functioning level at baseline. All the variables were comparable at baseline for the yoga and waitlist group.

## 7.2 SOCIAL COGNITION COMPOSITE SCORE (SCCS)

Mean & standard deviation for the groups at baseline and after one month is given in table-7.2. Data was found to be normally distributed and Repeated Measures ANOVA (RMANOVA) was applied with time and group as within and between factors respectively. RM ANOVA showed significant increase in Social Cognition Composite Score (SCCS) over time ($F= 26.89[1,34]$, $P<0.001$, partial eta squared=0.44) with a significant between group difference ($F=11.87[1]$, $P=0.002$, partial eta squared=0.25) favouring yoga intervention. There was significant interaction between time and group ($P<0.001$). Refer table-7.3 & Fig-7.2

**Table-7.1 Baseline and Sociodemographic data**

| Variables | YT(N=20) Mean(SD) | WL(N=20) Mean(SD) | t/$\chi^2$ | P |
|---|---|---|---|---|
| Age in Years | 32.70[7.0] | 31.45[6.0] | 0.6 | 0.55 |
| *Sex ratio, M: F | 13:07 | 14:06 | 0.11 | 0.73 |
| *Married: Single | 6:14 | 8:12 | 0.44 | 0.5 |
| Years of Education | 13.1[2.7] | 12.2[3.7] | 0.81 | 0.42 |
| Duration of illness | 9.2[6.0] | 7.1[4.5] | 1.2 | 0.21 |
| CGI illness severity | 4.7[1.0] | 5.1[0.7] | -1.47 | 0.14 |
| Antipsychotic dosage | 586.2[344.4] | 477.5[169.0] | 1.26 | 0.21 |
| SCCS score | 63.09[11.8] | 65.79[11.5] | -0.842 | 0.4 |
| Total SANS score | 51.11[12.0] | 45.59[14.0] | 1.27 | 0.21 |
| Total SAPS score | 31.21[13.5] | 28.59[13.6] | 0.48 | 0.63 |
| GSDS score | 43.42[11.0] | 40.88[9.2] | 0.3 | 0.76 |

*Ratios; YT-Yoga Therapy; WL-Wait List

SCCS-Social Cognition Composite Score; SANS-Scale for Assessing Negative Symptoms; SAPS-Scale for Assessing Positive Symptoms; GSDS-Groningen Social Disability Scale; CGI-Clinical Global Impression

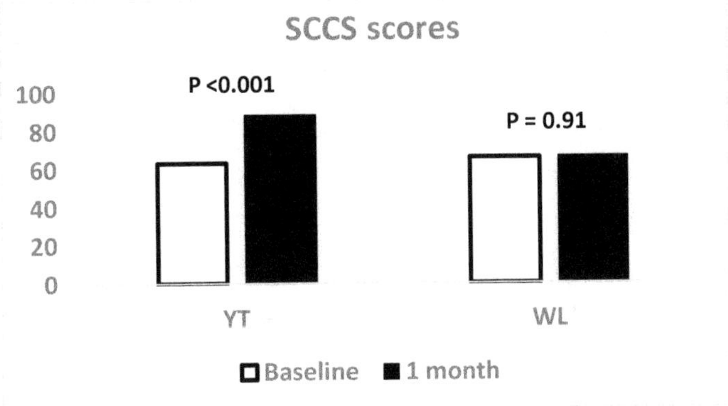


**Figure- 7.2 Change in Social Cognition Composite Score (SCCS) in percentage (Note: P value is for paired t test)**

## 7.3 TOTAL SANS SCORE

Mean & standard deviation for the groups at baseline and after one month is given in table-7.2. Data was found to be normally distributed and Repeated Measures ANOVA (RMANOVA) was applied with time and group as within and between factors respectively. RM ANOVA showed significant decrease in Total SANS Score over time (F= 142.13[1,33], P<0.001, partial eta squared=0.81) with a significant between group difference (F= 4.57[1], P=0.04, partial eta squared=0.12) favouring yoga intervention. There was significant interaction between time and group (P<0.001). (Refer table-7.3 & Fig-7.3)

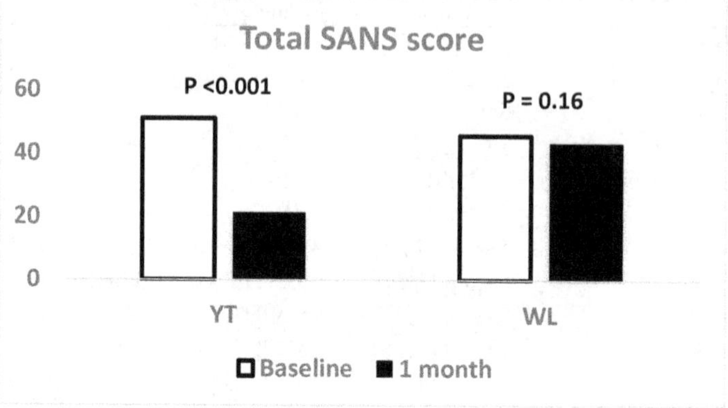


**Figure-7.3 Changes in Total SANS scores (Note: P value is for paired t test)**

## 7.4 TOTAL SAPS SCORE

Mean & standard deviation for the groups at baseline and after one month is given in table-7.2Data was found to be normally distributed and Repeated Measures ANOVA (RMANOVA) was applied with time and group as within and between factors respectively. RM ANOVA showed significant decrease in Total SAPS Score over time (F= 56.73[1,34], P<0.001, partial eta squared=0.62) with a non-significant between group difference (F= 1.97[1], P=0.16, partial eta squared=0.05). There was significant interaction between time and group (P=0.001). (Refer table-7.3 & Fig-7.4)

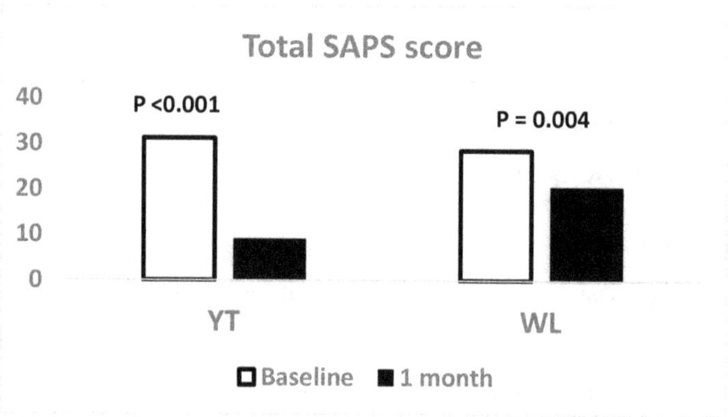


**Figure-7.4 Changes in Total SAPS scores (Note: P value is for paired t test)**

## 7.5 GSDS SCORE

Mean & standard deviation for the groups at baseline and after one month is given in table-7.2. Data was found to be normally distributed and Repeated Measures ANOVA (RMANOVA) was applied with time and group as within and between factors respectively. RM ANOVA showed significant increase in Total GSDS Score over time (F=78.20[1,34], P<0.001, partial eta squared=0.69) with a significant between group difference (F=4.82[1], P=0.03, partial eta squared=0.12) favouring yoga intervention. There was significant interaction between time and group (P<0.001). (Refer table-7.3 & Fig- 7.5)

## 7.6 BCATS (NEUROPSYCHOLOGICAL ASSESSMENTS

*Verbal Fluency Test (VFT)*

Mean & standard deviation for the groups at baseline and after one month is given in table-7.2. Data was found to be normally distributed and Repeated Measures ANOVA (RMANOVA) was applied with time and group as within and between factors respectively. RM ANOVA showed significant increase in VFT Score over time (F= 10.95[1,34], P=0.002, partial eta squared=0.24) with a non-significant between group difference (F= 3.19[1], P=0.08, partial eta squared=0.08) favouring yoga intervention. There was significant interaction between time and group (P=0.08). (Refer table-7.3 & Fig-7.6)

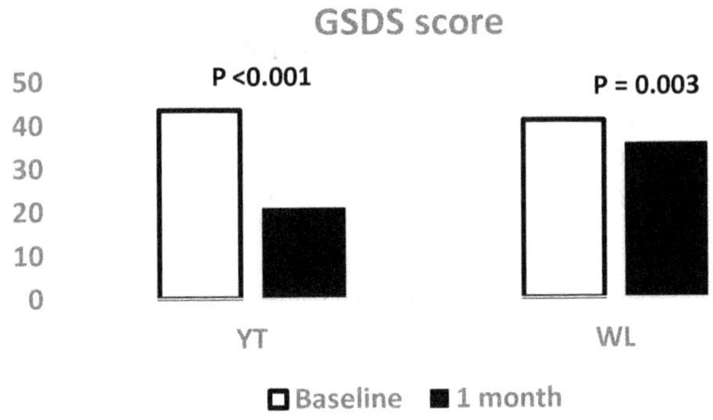


**Fig-7.5 Changes in GSDS scores (Note: P value is for paired t test )**

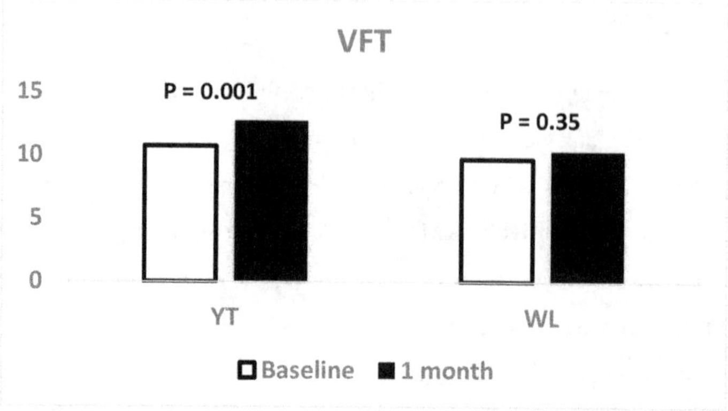


**Fig-7.6 Changes in VFT scores (Note: P value is for paired t test)**

***Digit symbol Substitution Test (DSST)***

Mean & standard deviation for the groups at baseline and after one month is given in table-7.2Data was found to be normally distributed and Repeated Measures ANOVA (RMANOVA) was applied with time and group as within and between factors respectively. RM ANOVA showed a non-significant decrease in time required to complete DSST over time (F= 2.93[1,34], P=0.9, partial eta squared=0.01) with a significant between group difference (F= 5.26[1], P=0.02, partial eta squared=0.13) favouring yoga intervention. There was no significant interaction between time and group (P=0.09). (Refer table-7.3 & Fig-7.7)

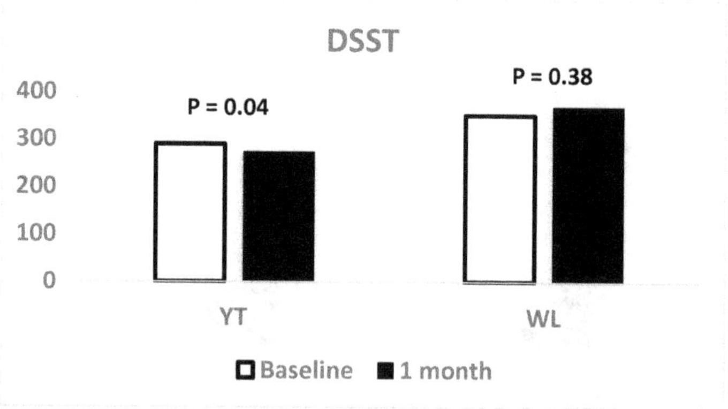


**Fig- 7.7 Changes in DSST scores (in Seconds) (Note: P value is for paired t test)**

*Colour trials test-B(CT-B)*

Mean & standard deviation for the groups at baseline and after one month is given in table-7.2. Data was found to be normally distributed and Repeated Measures ANOVA (RMANOVA) was applied with time and group as within and between factors respectively. RM ANOVA showed a non-significant decrease in time required to complete colour trials B over time (F= 2.0[1,33], P=0.01, partial eta squared=0.05) with a significant between group difference (F= 9.9[1], P=0.003, partial eta squared=0.23) favouring yoga intervention. There was no significant interaction between time and group (P=0.2). Refer table-7.3 & Fig-7.8

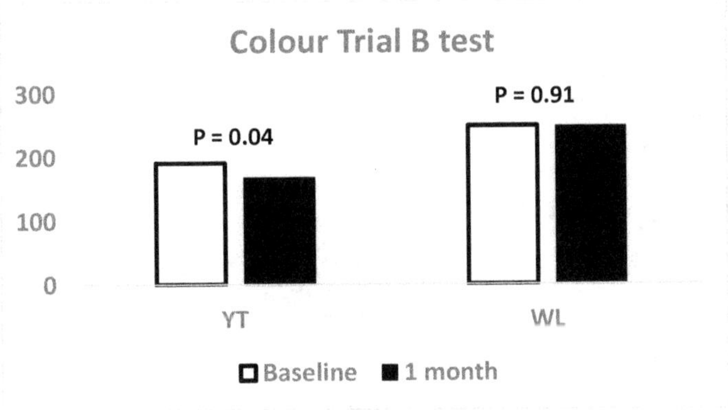


**Fig-7.8 Changes in Colour Trials B scores (in Seconds)**

**Table-7.2 Mean and Standard deviation of outcome variables**

| | YT(N=20) | | WL(N=20) | |
|---|---|---|---|---|
| Variables | Baseline Mean[SD] | 1 month Mean[SD] | Baseline Mean[SD] | 1 month Mean[SD] |
| SCCS | 63.09[11.8] | 88.00[10.2] | 65.79[11.5] | 66.14[10.5] |
| Total SANS | 51.11[12.0] | 21.17[8.3] | 45.59[14.0] | 43.18[13.3] |
| Total SAPS | 31.21[13.5] | 8.95[4.7] | 28.59[13.6] | 20.41[10.7] |
| GSDS | 43.42[11.0] | 20.63[9.2] | 40.88[9.2] | 35.41[8.6] |
| VFT | 10.73[3.2] | 12.68[3.4] | 9.7[2.8] | 10.29[2.7] |
| DSST | 290.05[61.9] | 272.15[65.8] | 351.11[131.71] | 368.82[150.2] |
| CT-B | 190.72[56.5] | 167.11[58.6] | 248.94[81.9] | 247.35[79.9] |

**Table-7.3 Results of RM-ANOVA for the outcome variables**

| | Within Group (time) | | Between Group (intervention) | |
|---|---|---|---|---|
| Variables (N) | F ($df_{time}$, $df_{error}$) | P value | F(df) | P value |
| SCCS (YT-19, WL-17) | 26.89[1,34] | <0.001 | 11.87[1] | 0.002 |
| Total SANS (YT-18, WL-17) | 142.13[1,33] | <0.001 | 4.57[1] | 0.04 |
| Total SAPS (YT-19, WL-17) | 56.73[1,34] | <0.001 | 1.97[1] | 0.16 |
| GSDS (YT-19, WL-17) | 78.20[1,34] | <0.001 | 4.82[1] | 0.03 |
| VFT (YT-19, WL-17) | 10.95[1,34] | 0.002 | 3.19[1] | 0.08 |
| DSST (YT-19, WL-17) | 2.93[1,34] | 0.9 | 5.26[1] | 0.02 |
| CT-B (YT-18, WL-17) | 2.0[1,33] | 0.1 | 9.9[1] | 0.003 |

SCCS-Social Cognition Composite Score; SANS-Scale for Assessing Negative Symptoms; SAPS-Scale for Assessing Positive Symptoms; GSDS-Groningen Social Disability Scale; VFT-Verbal Fluency Test; DSST-Digit Symbol Substitution Test; CT-B- Colour Trials B; YT-Yoga Therapy; WL-Wait List

Note: Numbers beside YT or WL represents the sample size analysed

## 7.7 MIRROR NEURON ACTIVITY(MNA)

**[with fNIRS in Left ventral Pre-Motor Cortex (LvPMC)]**

Mean and standard deviation of the BOLD signal for the Yoga Group, Waitlist Group and Combined (YT+WL) are given before intervention and after intervention in tables-7.4, 7.5, 7.6 respectively.

**Table- 7.4 Mean & Standard deviation of BOLD signal for yoga group before and after intervention**

| Conditions | Mean | SD |
|---|---|---|
| Pre_Static | 0.00004809 | 0.000373 |
| Pre_Action_obs | -0.00002691 | 0.000333723 |
| Pre_eAction_obs | -0.0000394 | 0.000081555 |
| Pre_perform | 0.00001087 | 0.000365725 |
| | | |
| Post_Static | -0.000013 | 0.000453122 |
| Post_Action_obs | -0.00023327 | 0.000467637 |
| Post_eAction_obs | 0.00024014 | 0.000499206 |
| Post_perform | 0.00018185 | 0.000373899 |

**Table-7.5 Mean & Standard deviation of BOLD signal for wait-list group before and after intervention**

| Conditions | Mean | SD |
|---|---|---|
| Pre_Static | -0.00022713 | 0.00038 |
| Pre_Action_obs | -0.00016347 | 0.00025766 |
| Pre_eAction_obs | 0.00038109 | 0.000571971 |
| Pre_perform | 0.00022941 | 0.000553726 |
| | | |
| Post_Static | 0.00005443 | 0.000322586 |
| Post_Action_obs | 0.00005581 | 0.000433092 |
| Post_eAction_obs | 0.00015522 | 0.000306423 |
| Post_perform | 0.00008785 | 0.000600126 |

**Table-7.6 Mean & Standard deviation of BOLD signal for yoga & wait-list group before and after intervention**

| Conditions | Mean | SD |
|---|---|---|
| Pre_Static_overall | -0.00015906 | .000370635 |
| Pre_Action_obs_overall | -0.00012991 | .000298104 |
| Pre_eAction_obs_overall | .00014898 | .000433141 |
| Pre_perform_overall | .00012391 | .000477240 |
| | | |
| Post_Static_overall | .00003419 | .000363494 |
| Post_Action_obs_overall | -.00001568 | .000390869 |
| Post_eAction_obs_overall | .00002174 | .000435942 |
| Post_perform_overall | -0.000088 | 0.00042 |

Pre-before yoga intervention: post-after yoga intervention Static-observing static image; Action_obs-observing goal directed action (video); eAction_obs- observing emotion embedded goal directed action (video) perform- motor task performance (opening & locking the lock)

*MNA calculation*

Presence of MNA was assessed by comparing the BOLD signal elicited by viewing a static image with that of goal directed video observation with or without emotion embedding and during motor task performance (opening &

locking a lock). MNA is said to be present if the BOLD signal in observing vs Goal directed action (video), Goal directed action emotion embedded (video) and motor task performance is significantly greater than the BOLD signal elicited by observing a static image.

All the data were non-normally distributed and hence Wilcoxon sign rank test was applied for comparison.

***Yoga Group (before intervention)***

*Observing static image vs Goal directed Action observation(video):*

There was no statistically significant difference in the BOLD signal between Observing static image vs Goal directed Action observation(video) and hence no MNA was present (P=0.57)

*Observing static image vs Goal directed Action observation (emotion embedded video):*

There was no statistically significant difference in the BOLD signal between Observing static image vs Goal directed emotion embedded action observation(video) and hence no MNA was present (P=0.81)

*Observing static image vs motor task performance:*

There was no statistically significant difference in the BOLD signal between Observing static image vs motor task performance and hence no MNA was present (P=0.73)

***Yoga Group (after intervention)***

*Observing static image vs Goal directed Action observation(video):*

There was no statistically significant difference in the BOLD signal between Observing static image vs Goal directed Action observation(video) and hence no MNA was present (P=0.08). P value is closer to significance level, but in the opposite direction (static >Action_obs)

*Observing static image vs Goal directed Action observation (emotion embedded video):*

There was no statistically significant difference in the BOLD signal between Observing static image vs Goal directed emotion embedded action observation(video) and hence no MNA was present (P=0.25)

*Observing static image vs motor task performance:*

There was no statistically significant difference in the BOLD signal between Observing static image vs motor task performance and hence no MNA was present (P=0.19)

***Wait List Group (before intervention)***

*Observing static image vs Goal directed Action observation(video):*

There was no statistically significant difference in the BOLD signal between Observing static image vs Goal directed Action observation(video) and hence no MNA was present (P=0.17)

*Observing static image vs Goal directed Action observation (emotion embedded video):*

There was statistically significant difference in the BOLD signal between Observing static image vs Goal directed emotion embedded action observation(video) and hence MNA was present (P=0.004) for this condition.

*Observing static image vs motor task performance:*

There was statistically significant difference in the BOLD signal between Observing static image vs motor task performance and hence MNA was present (P=0.006)

***Wait List Group (after intervention)***

*Observing static image vs Goal directed Action observation(video)*

There was no statistically significant difference in the BOLD signal between Observing static image vs Goal directed Action observation(video) and hence no MNA was present (P=0.56).

*Observing static image vs Goal directed Action observation (emotion embedded video)*

There was no statistically significant difference in the BOLD signal between Observing static image vs Goal directed emotion embedded action observation(video) and hence MNA was not present (P=0.004) for this condition.

*Observing static image vs motor task performance*

There was no statistically significant difference in the BOLD signal between Observing static image vs motor task performance and hence MNA was not present (P=0.86)

***Yoga Group + Wait List Group (before intervention)***

*Observing static image vs Goal directed Action observation(video)*

There was no statistically significant difference in the BOLD signal between Observing static image vs Goal directed Action observation(video) and hence no MNA was present (P=0.6).

*Observing static image vs Goal directed Action observation (emotion embedded video)*

There was statistically significant difference in the BOLD signal between Observing static image vs Goal directed emotion embedded action observation(video) and hence MNA was present (P=0.01) for this condition.

*Observing static image vs motor task performance*

There was statistically significant difference in the BOLD signal between Observing static image vs motor task performance and hence MNA was present (P=0.01)

***Yoga Group + Wait List Group (after intervention)***

*Observing static image vs Goal directed Action observation(video)*

There was no statistically significant difference in the BOLD signal between Observing static image vs Goal directed Action observation(video) and hence no MNA was present (P=0.87).

*Observing static image vs Goal directed Action observation (emotion embedded video)*

There was no statistically significant difference in the BOLD signal between Observing static image vs Goal directed emotion embedded action observation(video) and hence no MNA was present (P=0.44) for this condition.

*Observing static image vs motor task(performance)*

There was no statistically significant difference in the BOLD signal between Observing static image vs motor task performance and hence no MNA was present (P=0.49)

**Table-7.7 Wilcoxon Sign Rank test for Yoga Group**

| Conditions | N | P |
|---|---|---|
| Pre_Static-Action_obs | 15 | 0.57 |
| Pre_Static-eAction_obs | 12 | 0.81 |
| Pre_Static-perform | 14 | 0.73 |
| Post_Static-Action_obs | 15 | 0.08 |
| Post_Static-eAction_obs | 16 | 0.25 |
| Post_Static-perform | 16 | 0.19 |

Static-observing static image; Action_obs-observing goal directed action (video) eAction_obs- observing emotion embedded goal directed action (video) perform- motor task performance (opening & locking the lock)

**Table-7.8 Wilcoxon Sign Rank test for Wait-List Control Group**

| Conditions | N | P |
|---|---|---|
| Pre_Static-Action_obs | 15 | 0.17 |
| Pre_Static-eAction_obs | 16 | 0.004 |
| Pre_Static-perform | 15 | 0.006 |
| Post_Static-Action_obs | 16 | 0.56 |
| Post_Static-eAction_obs | 14 | 0.43 |
| Post_Static-perform | 15 | 0.86 |

**Table-7.9 Wilcoxon Sign Rank test for Yoga & Wait-List Control Group together**

| Conditions | N | P |
|---|---|---|
| Pre_Static-Action_obs_overall | 30 | 0.6 |
| Pre_Static-eAction_obs_overall | 28 | 0.01 |
| Pre_Static-perform_overall | 29 | 0.01 |
| | | |
| Post_Static-Action_obs_overall | 29 | 0.87 |
| Post_Static-eAction_obs_overall | 28 | 0.44 |
| Post_Static-perform_overall | 29 | 0.49 |

## 7.8 COMPARISON OF MNA BETWEEN BEFORE AND AFTER YOGA INTERVENTION

As there was no MNA detected for majority of the contrast, further analysis of comparing the MNA between before and after yoga was not done.

# Chapter 8.0
# DISCUSSION

# 8.0 DISCUSSION

## 8.1 SOCIAL COGNITION & MNA

This is one of the first studies exploring the role of yoga in social cognition. Previous studies have looked into the effect of yoga on Facial Emotion Recognition Deficit (FERD) in patients with schizophrenia. Previous studies (Jayaram et al., 2013) (R V Behere et al., 2011) have shown that yoga improves FERD in patients with schizophrenia. In this current study, social cognition is measured as a composite score which includes ToM (1$^{st}$ order and 2$^{nd}$ order), FERD, Social perception and Attribution Style (AS). Though we assessed AS, it was not included in the composite score calculation, as it gives information about the style of attribution but not of any numerical value that could be clubbed with other indices like ToM or social perception to arrive at a composite score for social cognition.

How does the overall social cognition improve with yoga still remains to be explored? Is it improving globally across all the domains of social cognition or is it a cascading effect of improvement in one/few domain(s) leading to improvement in other domains? We speculate that improvement in ToM could lead to improvement in other domains as well, as beliefs about self and others form the core for the social interactions and hence social cognition. Previous studies have also found ToM strongly correlating with the social functioning compared to other domains of social cognition and hence an important predictor for the same. Mirror Neuron Activity could also underpin the social cognition process as "imitation and being imitated" is one of the core processes of social interactions, though our study result does not support this speculation.

In our study, failure to detect the presence of MNA could be due to inadequate sample size. This is evident by the presence of MNA (overall MNA after merging both the intervention groups) in some of the conditions (contrast between static image observation and emotion embedded video observation and motor task performance - refer tables-7.8 & 7.9). This is one of the first studies using fNIRS to assess MNA the possibility of studying MNA with fNIRS and hence its utility with yoga intervention needs to be tested with adequate sample size.

## 8.2 CLINICAL SYMPTOMS AND SOCIAL FUNCTIONING

Results of this study is consistent with previous studies (Duraiswamy et al., 2007) (Varambally et al., 2012) (Jayaram et al., 2013) (R V Behere et al., 2011) which shows that yoga is useful in improving negative symptoms (measured by SANS) more than the positive symptoms (measured by SAPS). Improvement in the social functioning along with the negative symptoms following yoga suggest that these may be related to each other as evidenced by prior studies. Although some of the previous studies have shown improvement in positive symptoms, our study results did not show statically significant improvement.

## 8.3 NEUROPSYCHOLOGICAL TESTS

There was no significant improvement in any of the neuropsychological tests scores (VFT, DSST, CT-B) following yoga intervention. Previous studies with yoga intervention were mainly on healthy population. One of the consistent findings in majority of prior studies were improvement in attention (Gothe & McAuley, 2015).

## 8.4 POSSIBLE MECHANISMS OF ACTION OF YOGA

Yoga could possibly work by both bottom-up and top-down approaches - promoting relaxation through asana and pranayama, and mindfulness through chanting and positive resolution respectively. This dual effect of Yoga might well fit in with the dual processing theory of Social Cognition (Evans, 2008) , with mindfulness (yoga mediated) promoting controlled (reflective) processing and relaxation modulating the reflexive (automatic) processing.

Enhancement in reflective processing and modulated reflexive processing could also impact the hypo frontality and aberrant salience in patients with schizophrenia leading to improvement in clinical symptoms and hence social functioning.

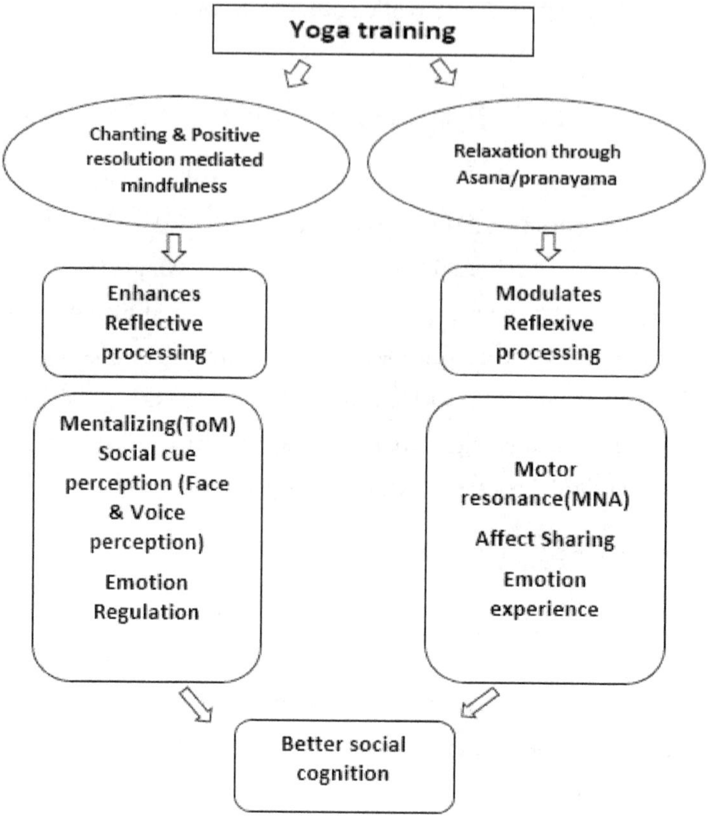


**Figure-8.1 Possible mechanisms of action of yoga**

# Chapter 9.0

# APPRAISAL

# 9.0 APPRAISAL

## 9.1 SUMMARY

In this thesis, we have attempted to demonstrate the utility of yoga in schizophrenia patients particularly on the social cognition aspect. Secondarily we also explored the possibility of using fNIRS for studying MNA, perhaps with a inadequate sample size. Another novelty is adding a motor task for eliciting MNA which may not be possible with other modalities like fMRI, TMS, etc.which are commonly used for studying MNA.

Improvement in overall social cognition and clinical symptoms including social functioning following yoga training is promising, as add-on yoga therapy might be more feasible compared to other available social cognition interventions like affect recognition training, cognitive enhancement therapy which are highly resource intensive.

## 9.2 CONCLUSION

One-month add-on yoga therapy improves social cognition, negative symptoms and social functioning. Add-on yoga therapy could also be considered along with available social cognition interventions, especially in Indian setup, as it is more culturally acceptable and feasible for its applications in clinical setup.

## 9.3 STRENGTHS OF THE STUDY

1) One of the first study on yoga intervention for social cognition in patients with schizophrenia

2) Throws light on novel methods of studying some of the aspects of social cognition like MNA with fNIRS; using motor task for assessing MNA

To our knowledge this is the second study which has used fNIRS for studying MNA in patient population.

3) Randomized trial design

## 9.4 LIMITATIONS OF THE STUDY

1) Samples were taken from both outpatient and inpatient department leading to heterogeneity and hence the inference may not be generalizable to any specific sample of patients.

2) Inspite of having taken all precautions to avoid any structured psychosocial co-interventions, we cannot rule out remote chances of inpatients improving just because of their social interactions with other patients, staff & treating team.

3) Only short-term effect of add-on yoga therapy was studied. Long term effect of add-on yoga therapy is not established which might have greater real-life utility for patients.

4) All yoga group subjects were given yoga intervention in a well-designed yoga centre, which may not be available for all patients in real life, considering the varied social profiles of patients and hence the results may not be ecologically valid until otherwise proven.

5) Being a physical activity based trial, the yoga therapist and subjects could not be blinded.

## 9.5 APPLICATION OF THE STUDY RESULTS

Considering the unavailability of effective pharmacotherapy and highly resource intensive psychosocial interventions for social cognitive deficits, add-on yoga therapy is an effective alternative for improving the clinical symptoms including social cognitive deficit in patients with schizophrenia.

Utility of add-on yoga therapy for cognitive deficit could possibly be extended to other psychiatric disorders like Autism and bipolar disorders in the future.

## 9.6 SUGGESTIONS FOR FUTURE WORK

Future studies could focus on the following aspects

1) Long term effect of add-on yoga therapy on social cognition

2) Social interaction based active control group could be compared with yoga therapy group, to avoid the confounding related to social interactions leading to chance improvement in social cognition

3) MNA could be studied with larger sample size and MNA's relation to social cognition could be explored

4) Since logistics- especially the travel distance and the negative symptoms form the major hurdle for participating and sustaining regular yoga practices, community based yoga training could be explored for easy adherence to regular yoga practices.